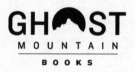

Dr. and Mrs. Guinea Pig

Present

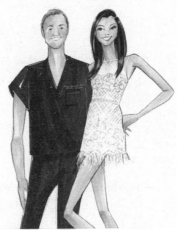

The Only Guide You'll *Ever* Need to the Best Anti-Aging Treatments

by

Heather Dubrow and Terry Dubrow M.D., F.A.C.S.

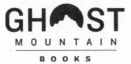

GH◯ST

MOUNTAIN

BOOKS

Published in Los Angeles, California, by Ghost Mountain Books, Inc.

ISBN:
Print 9781939457554
EPub 9781939457547
Mobi 9781939457530

Cover Photo: Rod Foster/Gigasavvy.com
Cover Design: Longerday.com
Interior Design and production: Dovetail Publishing Services

Dedications

I dedicate this book to my doctor, my best friend, and the love of my life. They happen to all be the same person. Terry, thank you for twenty years of love, laughter, and coproducing our four amazing children. Even though I don't like rodents, I am happy to be your guinea pig for life.

—Heather

I'd like to dedicate this book to my favorite experimental subject of all time, the cutest lab animal there is, my wife and life partner, Heather Dubrow. You have graciously (albeit with some minor kicking and screaming) allowed me to throw everything I have at you so we find the best, no-BS solutions to this crazy and often uncharted world of health, wellness, and beauty. Between you thinking everything works and me believing nothing works, we have created the ultimate no-nonsense guide to aging gracefully, designed to help everyone look better and feel better, no matter how old they are. No doctor has ever had a more intelligent, supportive, loving wife, friend, and laboratory rat. I love you, Honyi.

—Terry

Contents

Acknowledgments

Way too many people to thank and brevity is not one of our strong suits, but we will try . . .

Thank you to our children, Nicky, Max, Kat, and Coco. We love you so much and appreciate how you pretended to be interested as we talked endlessly about experiments, treatments, and products during dinner these last two years .

Thank you to everyone at Ghost Mountain Books, especially Jay McGraw for seeing our vision and Lisa Clark for being our editor and cheerleader and always making sure we stayed on course. Karen Moline, one of the coolest, smartest gals we have ever known, your expertise and guidance have been invaluable. Also thanks to Andrea McKinnon and Carly Stratton for your tireless efforts to bring our book to life.

Thank you to our agents Lance Klein, Mel Berger, and Ryan McNeily at WME for always supporting us and our crazy ideas.

Kelly Kline, Stephanie Massey, and Dawn Hawley, thank you for lending your incredible talents to our book. Your expert knowledge and tips not only make us look good in real life, but added such a special perspective for our readers.

Thank you to our unbelievable assistant, Natalie Puche. Not only are you one of the smartest, sweetest people we know, but also a beautiful girl, inside and out. You are a huge part of making our world work and we are eternally grateful for you.

Note to Readers

The anecdotes in this book are used to illustrate common issues and problems that we have encountered, and do not necessarily portray specific people or situations. No real names have been used. This book is comprised of the opinions and ideas of its authors and is meant solely for general informational and entertainment purposes on the subjects addressed in the book. The ideas and concepts in this book are not intended to diagnose, treat, cure, or prevent any medical, health, mental, physical, psychological, or psychiatric problem or condition, nor are they meant to substitute for professional advice of any kind. Specific questions and decisions about treatments should be made in partnership with your health care provider.

Health information changes rapidly. Therefore, some information within this book may be out of date or even possibly inaccurate and/or erroneous. The reader should consult his or her medical, health, psychological, or other competent professional before adopting any of the concepts in this book or drawing inferences from it. The content of this book, by its very nature, is general, whereas each reader's situation is unique. Therefore, as with all books of this nature, the purpose is to provide general information rather than address individual situations, which books by their very nature cannot do.

The author and publisher specifically disclaim all responsibility for, and are not liable for, any liability, loss, or risk, personal or otherwise, which is incurred as a consequence, directly or indirectly, of the use and application of any of the contents of this book.

Any and all product names referenced within this book are trademarks of their respective owners. None of these owners have sponsored, authorized, endorsed, or approved this book in any way. Unless otherwise noted, the authors are in no way affiliated with any brands or products recommended in this book. Always read all information provided by the manufacturers' product labels before using their products. We are not responsible for claims made by product manufacturers. The statements made in this book have not been evaluated by the U.S. Food and Drug Administration.

Introduction

Are you feeling and looking your age, and not happy about it? Fret no more! This book is going to become your anti-aging bible. We're going to cover all the available techniques and treatments from brand new to time-tested, from perfectly legal to frankly illegal, from the simple to the outrageous. This will not only allow you to devise the very best home anti-aging plan, but it will also provide you with the tools and knowledge you need in order to seek out the right procedures and professionals when appropriate.

Allow me to rewind to when we first met, on a blind date in 1996. I had moved out to California from a small town in Westchester County, New York. My mother had always been into excellent skincare, but there wasn't a lot of talk about plastic surgery, except to comment about the occasional nose job done on one of my sixteen-year-old classmates. It was an absolute culture shock when I moved to Los Angeles! I had majored in musical theater when I got my bachelor's degree at Syracuse University, and instead of moving to New York City to hopefully end up on Broadway as I had originally planned, I got sidetracked by a TV show and ended up in La-La Land to be a television and film actress. I worked incredibly hard, went on more auditions than I care to remember, and was excited for my big break with a recurring role on the WB show *Life with Roger*.

This was about the time I met Terry, and we really hit it off. I could tell from his professional scrutiny that he appreciated my brains *and* my figure, even though on our first date I was wearing a little black dress that sort of smushed down my breasts, which were naturally a small D before those four kids sucked the life out of them . . . but I'm getting ahead of myself. Terry watched my show the following week to see me in action. As soon as the episode was over, my phone rang.

"Wow," he said. "You're a really good actress. And forgive me for not noticing, but you've got exceptional breasts. I had *no* idea from the dress you were wearing."

1

I smiled at the phone. It was so cute how he said that. Except then he moved in for the kill.

"But did you know that when you make that squinty *face*," he went on, "you get these deep lines between your eyebrows?"

My jaw dropped and I thought, holy crap, that was *so rude*. I immediately said, "No, I don't!"

"Yes, you do," he said, ignoring my protest. "Come to my office whenever you like. If I gave you a little bit of Botox, it would just soften those lines and then you'll never get wrinkles there."

"I can't believe you would say something like that to me," I replied, thinking to myself that he was just an arrogant so-and-so and what a shame because I really liked him!

Well, when the show was next on TV, of course I was watching. I looked at myself on the small screen and realized, *ugh*, Terry was right! I hadn't even noticed those lines before and now I couldn't stop staring at them.

So I went into his office for Botox . . . and the rest is history!

One happy marriage, four amazing children, and seven reality shows later, here we are. Terry has become one of the best-known and successful plastic surgeons in America, and I am still acting, appearing on *The Real Housewives of Orange County*, hosting the *Botched: Post-Op* show, singing at events, doing my top-rated podcast on PodcastOne, running a skincare company, supervising our household, overseeing the crazy building of a new house, raising our kids, and writing this book with Terry. It's nuts, but I can't think of anything else I'd rather be doing!

Turning back the clock is a constant thread in our community. Yes, we all know that everyone ages; fifty is the new forty, or even thirty, right? Some people, like fine wine, age better than others. But because aging is a complicated process, most people think that treating its effects must be complicated, too. That isn't true. The secret to great skin is both getting it *and* maintaining it.

Then why do some people, including celebrities, look and feel so much better and younger than others their same age? What are their secrets? Is it the luck of the genetic draw? Potent new drugs or treatments? Fabulous skincare products? Multiple visits to talented plastic surgeons?

The answer is simple: *Yes.* It's all of the above. Never before have we lived in an era where so much is available to those who search it out—so much that can thwart and even, at times, reverse the aging process.

My friends, as well as perfect strangers who know me from TV, come to me with their anti-aging questions because there's such an information overload about skincare that they have no idea what's real and what's bogus. They know I'm a down-to-earth person, dealing with the same skincare and aging issues that everybody else is dealing with. They know I'll be blunt with them about their understandable confusion that has led them, as it has most consumers, to choose skincare products and more in-depth treatments without really understanding what might work best—or what won't work at all.

After years of fielding these questions, Terry and I knew there was a real need for this book. Here are the four reasons why we decided to write it:

1. To end confusion

Terry: Many of the patients who come to me are overwhelmed by their options, or they've been seriously disappointed with botched procedures they had. They don't want to look as if they could have entered the witness protection program. They want to look like *themselves*—only better—yet they are continually pushed to undergo procedures that won't do the best job for their needs. How can I best help them figure out what to do?

2. To share our wealth of knowledge

Terry: Our mission is to differentiate the con jobs of the health, wellness, and beauty industries from what actually works. Heather and I have tried practically every anti-aging product out there, and we love being Dr. and Mrs. Guinea Pig—on the E! network's show *Good Work*, and with our friends and my patients. Heather is a savvy consumer and I am a savvy surgeon with access to all the newest and most advanced devices and anti-aging procedures. We want to tell you everything you need to know about how to turn back the clock—things your friends don't know and your doctors and plastic surgeon aren't going to tell you! Even more important, if you want to have surgery, you can do it safely—once you read everything I have to tell you in chapter 6.

3. To save you time and money

We believe everyone should have effective skincare that doesn't cost a fortune. This book will teach you what works and what doesn't.

4. To destigmatize anti-aging treatments and plastic surgery

Heather: Everyone thinks I've had my whole face done. Botox, yes. Filler, once—I got Sculptra when I was über-thin because my face was showing it. A facelift, no. A new nose, no, even though I have a bump in the middle so I always take pictures from one side to reduce its appearance. I asked Terry to shave it off and he refused—he told me that, no, it gives me character, and I have to admit that he's right. But if I get to the point where I feel I need it or want it, sign me right up!

As for Botox, I love it even though I use it sparingly—believe me, I want my children to know when I'm angry! I've never had any problems discussing it. Why would I be ashamed? I love that the stuff works so well and I love appreciating Terry's skill when he does the injections. (That is, of course, one of the great perks of being married to a plastic surgeon!) Still, my friends and fellow actresses were shocked when I did an interview for *InStyle* magazine a few years ago, and when the journalist asked me what the weirdest thing was that I kept in my refrigerator, I told her it was Botox. Just in case I needed it.

Talking about it is only a big deal if *you* make it a big deal! That brings us to a very important point: we know that if you *can't* talk about your anti-aging treatments, you are much less likely to get the best possible advice. This is especially needed if you're tempted to walk into one of those storefront laser centers with "deals" advertised in their windows.

Terry: The more comfortable we are talking about any procedures, the more comfortable we are talking about the *problems* that can occur. It's so important to have a healthy dose of paranoia about any treatment and especially about elective cosmetic surgery.

This issue is very dear to my heart. About two years before I was chosen to be on *Botched*, I became totally disillusioned with the plastic surgery business. I felt that all my surgical skills were going to waste; I had gone from saving lives to being burned out. But since the show started, I've been reinvigorated by my love for helping people who really need helping. I see people who had thought their lives were over become transformed once they're un-botched. And that is what a surgeon's life should be about. When you fix people's appearances, you make them happy. When you help them make informed decisions, you make them happy, too.

How to Use This Book

To get the best possible results, our philosophy is to start slowly. First, try the least invasive treatments and procedures and see how they work. If you're not satisfied, it's time to think about moving on to more invasive procedures with proven results. We've structured the book to follow this concept. Here's how we've laid it out:

Part I—Heather's Hollywood Handbook of Anti-Aging Tricks: Makeup and Hair How-To's will show you how to stylishly and easily turn back the clock.

Part II—Products, Treatments, and Procedures Guide is your go-to guide for all things skincare and treatment, from over-the-counter to surgery.

Part III—Dr. and Mrs. Guinea Pig Ratings shows you what works *best* for any skincare and anti-aging treatments you're considering.

Part IV—The Good, the Bad, and the Crazy takes you on a tour of the latest, craziest, and sometimes surprisingly helpful hippest, hottest, newest procedures. If it's out there, you can bet someone in Hollywood is doing it!

With the tools in this book, you will learn how to feel and look your very best, regardless of your age. We want to make sure you *never* get botched. No one should strive to be "perfect," because that is an impossible goal. As Heather says, "When you feel good, you *look* good."

So read on. Dr. and Mrs. Guinea Pig are here to help!

PART
I

*Heather's Hollywood Handbook of
Anti-Aging Tricks: Makeup and
Hair How-To's*

CHAPTER

1

Heather's Hollywood Anti-Aging Makeup Manual

Being an actress is hard work. You see the end result—the movie or TV show, the red carpet, the photographs, the fans, the nice salary—but what you don't see is the effort that went into making it look effortless. Acting is as much about competition and rejection as it is about landing those great parts. And, especially for women, it's about being judged on your looks. As in scrutinized, criticized, laughed at, mocked, nitpicked, and savaged, especially in the super-ageist Hollywood where you're toast once you hit a certain age and your face starts to show the very natural results of the very natural aging process. (This is the Hollywood where, you might recall, Nicole Kidman once played a brain surgeon, in the film *Days of Thunder*, when she was only twenty-three—she must have been some kind of medical school prodigy to pull that one off!)

The new technology, although great for viewers, isn't helping the issue! High- definition TV is a friend to no one over the age of sixteen. The screen shows every nook and cranny of your skin. I swear at some point our newscasters will be fourteen, because they will be the only ones that look good under a microscope!

I think it's utterly ridiculous that actresses aren't supposed to have laugh lines because we're happy or frown lines because, well, some people get on our nerves and we can't help the frowning! But I don't see this attitude changing anytime soon. So, like my friends and colleagues in the business, I learned early on how to grow a thick skin and not let the hurt show.

When I joined the cast of *The Real Housewives of Orange County*, however, I realized it wasn't so thick after all. The fans of reality TV, through blogs and social media, are very vocal about how the cast members look scene to scene, episode to episode. This isn't scripted TV with a director of photography and a crew working to make you look perfect. This is a documentary-style show that has a raw, real feel to make you feel as though you are there. Unfortunately, we don't always look great, even if we *did* look great that day! It was very difficult for me to deal with the scrutiny for the first couple of years, but gradually, thank goodness, I got over it. I'm happy with how I look. I'm grateful that I can access so much good advice about how to look this way, too.

I learned an awful lot about how life doesn't happen in high def. When I want to look my best, I go for the opposite of what Hollywood glam is supposed to be. I am not going to be the woman who had her makeup artist come over and duct-tape the back of her neck to give herself an instant, temporary facelift before we shot our scenes. Yes, I've seen this with my own eyes!

In other words, my anti-aging makeup philosophy is simple: *less is more.* So this is what I wear everyday, when I'm just going about my innumerable errands: *absolutely nothing.*

Okay, maybe I'll add a little lip gloss, but it's only to keep my lips hydrated, not because I feel the need for color. If you have clean, healthy, well-hydrated skin, you don't need to wear much makeup at all. And certainly not a mask of thick foundation that will call attention to the parts of your face you're trying to cover up!

That sure wasn't me back in the 1980s when I was growing up. It was all about big, bold hair; big, bold colors for my eyes and lips; and way, way too much makeup! I started wearing lip gloss in the sixth grade, like practically everybody else in my class, and during junior high, my mom would let me wear a little blush for special occasions. By high school, I went for it. Except the au courant look we all went for at the time was this weird rainbow technique; the inner of your eye was one color, and then the middle section was one color, and the end was another color. (I absolutely blame my sister for this . . . and Duran Duran.) I really thought I was on point with my scrunchie spray waterfall bangs. Then, in my short-lived goth phase, it was all about black lipstick and pale faces for me and my sister.

My mother was smart. Her philosophy was that as long as it's not something that's permanent that we'd regret later, go ahead and experiment. And that's how I feel about makeup now—go ahead and experiment. Have fun. Try new looks. Don't get stuck in a rut. Then wash it all off and start all over again. With *less*!

Because I started my career in the theater where I had to do my own makeup, and because I've worked with so many great makeup artists over the years, I've learned a lot of their tricks. Few people believe this, but I do my own makeup when I'm filming, even for *The Real Housewives of Orange County*. The only exception is if the lights are really hot and my face is going to look different, I know the show's makeup artists have different kinds of foundation and other products to let my skin look its best. Otherwise, I like doing my own makeup. I like playing around with colors on my cheeks and eyes; I actually find it kind of cathartic. And I now have a couple of go-to looks as my signatures that I can pull off super-fast.

These are my favorite makeup tips, along with the first of several bonus tips in this chapter from Hollywood makeup artist Stephanie Massie:

1. You can get great advice at department store makeup counters. Take advantage of them!

Makeup is a skill like anything else, so all you need is a bit of practice and a good teacher. Department stores have trained makeup artists at the counters, most of whom will do your makeup for free. Or you can go when you know you have the budget to buy a new lipstick or eye shadow so you don't feel any pressure to buy a lot. You can ask the makeup artist to first do one side and then have you do the other so you can see how to replicate their look.

2. Hire a pro to come to you.

If you live in a major city and you do want to hire a professional but don't know how to find one, go to www.theglamapp.com, where you can book a

Stephanie Tip: I've found that many women get discouraged with makeup because they take products home and aren't sure how to use them properly. That's why I think they need a professional opinion at the makeup counter. We're so hard on ourselves, and I know a lot of women are afraid to make a mistake and look ridiculous. I always tell women that there are no "rules" when it comes to makeup. I can do my whole face with my fingers super quick with cream-based products. I put the eye shadow crayon on, rub it in, and throw some mascara on and maybe a lipstick and I'm done. Everyone thinks I spent forty minutes on my makeup and it probably took three! An expert can teach you how to do the same in no time.

makeup artist (and hair and nail stylist, too) who will come to your home or office. It's fabulous for when your time is limited and you want to "wow" at a special event. And you'll learn lots of tricks, too.

One of the big advantages to hiring a makeup pro is that they'll give you ideas you might never have thought of, and they'll know what will look good with your skin tone. The whole point is to ask questions and try new things. Even if you have found the perfect red lipstick, there will always be new formulations that might be just as yummy.

With a makeup artist, try not to control the situation. Avoid comments like "I always wear blue eyeliner" or "I don't like blush." Their opinions about blue eyeliner and blush may be a whole lot better than yours. Or at least different. Trust them to know what they're doing!

3. Don't get stuck in a makeup rut.

Even though I have a go-to look for my makeup, I definitely experiment and try to change it up.

Some women really get stuck in their makeup rut, wearing the same colors by the same brands they wore in high school, even though their lives are much different. They may be afraid of color, or don't want to be judged, or aren't sure what to do, so they stick to the same old same old, or they're so overwhelmed by choices that they end up making no choices at all!

I understand that, really, because I'm comfortable with my "look." Am I in a rut? Not really, because every few months, I take my time browsing in Sephora, just to keep up with the new products. Not that I'd jump on every trend, especially if I know they won't suit me. Remember when Chanel's Vamp came out? It was a deep, blood red, and it looked great on models and cadavers, but not on me. But it was such a popular color that I got Vamp nail polish. *Voila!* On trend, and still using my regular palette on my face.

My advice about makeup ruts is to realize that makeup is one of the cheapest ways you can instantly change your appearance and make yourself feel good. I've seen women put on a brand-new lipstick color and they immediately look ten years younger. It's amazing when that happens!

If you have a friend defensively stuck in a rut, a nice gesture is to book a makeover for you both. That way, it's not too obvious that you're trying to help. For someone who wants a change but doesn't know what to do, get her a gift certificate for a brand with a beauty bar or makeup artists at the department store counter, and go with her for her do-over. Or ask her to go with you when you're makeup shopping and buy her a small item. My friends are much more likely to use a gift than something they'd buy themselves.

Also, don't throw out your "gift with purchase" items! They're a great way to experiment with something different.

4. Not all makeup brands are created equal, and this is one category where you do get what you pay for.

Since I've experimented with so much makeup, I realized that the better brands *are* worth it, especially for lips and eyes. The colors stay true and they last so much longer that they become more cost-effective over the long run.

5. Use good lighting.

Lighting is such an important part of makeup application—too dark and done with a heavy hand, and you end up looking much older; too soft, and you won't be able to see where you need extra coverage, making your skin look veiny and splotchy. Experiment with lighting the same way you experiment with makeup and brushes, and recognize how different lighting changes how your makeup looks. That's why less is more, and understated neutrals will keep you from having to worry about an intense shade turning on you. I use one of those close-up magnifying mirrors with the halo of light around it, and I glance back and forth between that and the larger bathroom mirror. Be careful about the mirror setting—some of them cast a pink or warm glow that changes the way your makeup looks in real life. Avoid that and use the brightest, clearest light instead. *Then* check it in another room.

Lighting is also important when you're planning to experiment—try a new color *before* you go somewhere special. At the reunion for *Real Housewives* a couple of years ago, I was wearing a stunning blue Victoria Beckham dress and had a sleek new hairdo. I had bought a new Tom Ford eye shadow palette that included a gorgeous navy blue, so I thought it would look perfect in my crease. I did one last check before I went to the set, and in still photos (which I took *a lot* of!) the makeup looked like perfection. However, when I was on the set under the very bright lights covered with different color "gels" to create atmosphere, it was a whole different ballgame! When I watched the show, I was horrified to see that it was so flipping blue under the light I looked like Mimi from *The Drew Carey Show*. Lesson learned—the hard way!

6. Don't use heavy foundation as a mask—it's so aging!

Makeup is fun; I love being playful with my makeup. And I love washing off anything I thought was going to make me look young, but didn't. Too much makeup will *always* age you. As with good skincare, or even plastic surgery, you want to use makeup to enhance your looks, not make you look fake, brittle, or plastic.

If you like foundation, use a subtle hand. You'll protect your skin from the sun (which is *guaranteed* to age you) and you'll look polished. Trust me on this—women who swear by their "natural" look have spent hours in the bathroom doing all sorts of makeup tricks to look "natural." I have much better things to do with my time! And I'm sure you do, too.

How to Look More Youthful with Makeup—Go Minimal

When we're younger, we want to look older, and when we're older, we want to look younger, right? Whenever I post pictures of myself without makeup, what do I hear? "Wow, you look so much younger!" Let your skin breathe. Give it the glow from a healthy diet and regular exercise and drinking lots of water—not from a ton of makeup!

Make sure you tailor your makeup to the occasion. When I go to a party or a special event in Hollywood, I'll do a dramatic face—lots of fake lashes, darker eye shadow, more intense lip color; my clothes will be sparkly and my heels so high my bunions will be screaming the next day. (Yes, this is a sad remnant from cheerleading and dance days!) My daughters love when I'm all glammed-out, but my son thinks it's too much. He prefers a more natural look. (Future dates be warned!) For a daytime meeting, I'll put on a very sheer palette, with pale lips, a hint of blush, and a sheer caramel eye shadow because I want to look light and fresh; my outfit will be something simple like a black leather pencil skirt, blouse, and a simple pump.

Stephanie Tip: To streamline your makeup routine, ask yourself what's important to you that day. Do you want to look rosy, or wide awake, or hide some wrinkles, and so on. For a little punch, a sweep of blush on your cheeks and eyelids will give a hint of color. If you have amazing skin, all you need is a lip color and mascara. When I'm wearing lipstick, it looks like I'm wearing a full face of makeup. If you like a little foundation coverage, then you're good to go with just lip balm and an eye shadow cream pencil. Also, look for multitasking products. Everyone's so stuck on, "Oh, that is for eyebrows only. You can't use that as an eyeliner . . ." But you can!

Here's our best product advice:

Makeup for Your Skin

Primer

Back in the olden days when I started paying attention to makeup, there was an under-eye primer that, after you put it on, was so tight that if you just stood there you looked great . . . but as soon as you made any facial expressions, your whole face cracked! You looked like you were eighty years old and about to keel over. Not a good look.

Maybe that's why I've never been a huge fan of primers, which is an undercoat you put on over your moisturizer and before your foundation. A lot of my friends love them, but I've found them to be very drying because many of them are designed to minimize oil and shine, which usually isn't needed once you're past a certain age. They can accentuate pores and often have a white base that can make you look ghostly in photos.

Best to go for blur products as primers, which you will read about in the section on pores in chapter 4. These are usually silicone-based and are like a spackle that minimizes pores and temporarily fills in fine lines and wrinkles. A blur product is like Photoshop for your skin. If you use a good one, you don't need foundation on top of it.

Foundation

I only wear foundation when I'm being filmed, because it can be incredibly aging. It's especially hard for older women and people with problem skin to give up their "coverage," but they should!

Foundation is the descendent of the thick pancake makeup Max Factor (yes, he was a real person!) developed for Hollywood in the 1930s, when the lights on the sets were incredibly hot and actors needed heavy-duty coverage. There are now a gazillion foundations, but the purpose is still the same: to give you some coverage and even out your skin tone. You want to see the natural beauty of your skin; foundation is supposed to color-correct your skin tone, not hide it from the world!

When I have to wear foundation, I wear a "color correcting" (CC) cream that has a tint and SPF and gives you a natural, even look while letting the beauty of your skin show through. If you're trying to kick the foundation habit, try a tinted moisturizer or a CC cream instead. It will give you some coverage, and if you get one with SPF, even better. For an even more sheer look, mix a bit of your foundation or your tinted moisturizer in the palm of your hand with a bit of sunscreen. You'll get more sun protection and still look good.

If you like foundation, there are two crucial steps to follow:

❖ *Get the right match.* Go to a department store and ask for samples, because you need to test it on your skin—not in the harsh fluorescent store lights but outside in daylight and/or in your office or home, where you'll be wearing it the most. (If they don't have samples, bring a little ziplock bag and pour a tiny bit in to test out later.) Keep trying until you find the hue that seamlessly blends into your own skin. It isn't easy!

❖ *Blend, blend, blend!* I use my fingers, but a lot of pros like the little white disposable sponges you can find at any drugstore. Be sure to blend under your neck, too; nothing is more aging than a visible line where the foundation stops.

Stephanie Tip: There are three ways to apply foundation: with your fingers, a sponge, and a brush. Some people use a combination of the three. With a brush, use a buffing motion as well to make sure it's well blended and to make it look like a flawless finish.

Contouring

Contouring as a trend is way out of control. It will not only make you look deliberately fake, but it can draw attention to your face for all the wrong reasons. Done incorrectly (as it often is), contouring is *instantly* aging, as it can't cover lines and wrinkles. Recently, I saw a friend who is usually on-point, but this time, her contouring was comical; it looked like stripes on her face! You want people to notice you, *not* your makeup.

If you feel it's a must, choose a light bronzer for the contour; it's much harder to overdo. Also, there are many YouTube tutorials demonstrating contouring techniques for an extremely polished look. They're a great help *if* you know what you're doing. Trust me, this is a skill that needs a *lot* of practice!

Concealer

No one has perfect skin all the time, which is why we use concealers. I love my CC cream by Kate Somerville. It's super light and has an SPF, but it's still opaque enough to cover any imperfections or under-eye circles.

Another secret is my magic eraser, Camouflage from glō-minerals. It's a very inexpensive oil-free concealer you can get at beauty supply stores. I like the color "natural" and it seems to work on most Caucasian skin types. It comes in a little pot and instantly erases my red spots and dark circles. You can even layer it on top of your foundation to reapply in the evening. Be sure to apply it with your ring finger and gently dab it on. The less you use and the less you touch it when applying, the better.

Powder

When I'm filming, I have to wear foundation, so I love a good translucent high-definition powder as well. It sets the foundation, prevents shine (which is death when you're on TV!), helps keep it true to its color, and allows it to last longer. Most of all, a high-def powder doesn't reflect light, which is crucial when you're shooting or having your photo taken.

My go-to powder is from Le Métier de Beauté. It's a powder foundation, but I love the color (#3) and the texture. I don't want it to be too thick or drying so I mix it with MAKE UP FOR EVER's HD Microfinish Powder. That's what I use to set my foundation, and it only takes two seconds to give me that really beautiful finish. You only want a dusting, and mixing the two powders together makes it even lighter.

Your Makeup Is Only as Good as Your Tools!

You know those little brushes or sponges that come with eye shadows? Toss them. Immediately. They don't work and they can really yank and irritate the skin on your eyes.

Just like you need good knives in the kitchen, you need a good set of makeup brushes. They come with different types of hair and at varying prices, and the best thing to do is find some that fit comfortably in your hand so you actually use them. They make makeup application so much easier, quicker, and more precise.

What you need: a small eye shadow brush, a crease brush, a small slanted brush for eyebrow powder, an eyeliner brush if you use liquid liner, a blush/bronzer brush, and a large puff for powder and/or bronzer.

Don't forget to clean them regularly—otherwise they're havens for bacteria and dirt. It's cost-effective to buy a brand like Cinema Secrets professional-grade brush cleaner, pour it into a smaller clear spray bottle, and then just spray your brushes. Wipe the excess cleaner off with a tissue or paper towel and let them air-dry overnight. Never store wet brushes upright, as the water can run into the handle and cause it to warp or crack.

Stephanie Tip: One of the biggest mistakes you can make as you get older is to use too much powder and drying products and not enough moisture. I usually apply powder with a brush, but for a more glamorous look, use a sponge or puff, then buff it off with a brush.

Once a week, I wash my brushes and condition them with shampoo. Just make a diluted solution in a bowl, dip them in, swish around, and rinse. It makes them last longer and they'll look brand new.

Just be sure to blend it well. If you've ever seen a photo of a celebrity with visible white streaks under her eyes, it's because the makeup artist forgot to dust off the powder. Don't let that be you!

Blush and Bronzer

My mother always said, "Never leave the house without blush on or you will run into everyone!" Nothing says sick looking or old like a sallow complexion. Even back in the day, women would pinch their cheeks to give them a healthy glow. The key here is *subtlety*. Too much blush or bronzer looks fake. If you're not using foundation (hint!), then your cheeks will naturally have a bit of color to them, no matter what your skin tone.

Even though I am naturally pale skinned, I appreciate the effect of a light bronzer. It's a great way to warm up the skin instead of contouring. Apply it in a number-three pattern starting at the forehead. This will avoid the fake, painted-on "stripe" look.

My favorite is Tom Ford's bronzing powder in #02 Terra. It's expensive but it lasts forever, and a little goes a long way. Stay away from cream formulas, as they can be hard to blend, and as soon as you start rubbing, your cheeks get all red and then you can't tell what your blush looks like and you have to start all over again!

Makeup for Your Eyes

Eye Shadow

Long gone are those days of my rainbow-colored eyes! Neutrals are the way to go. Makeup is intended to enhance our natural looks. Using a neutral palette allows our features to be the star. You want people to notice you, not your makeup.

Eyeliner and Eye Pencils

A little bit of eyeliner can make your eyes pop and look bigger; it takes a bit of practice, so take your time learning. I prefer a liquid eyeliner on my upper eyelids because it gives me a nice, smooth line, hides tiny bumps or irregularities, and glides over skin that's getting more crepey with age. If

Stephanie Tip: For a neutral palette that works on all skin tones, I like MAC's x15 Warm Neutral Palette or Urban Decay's original Naked Palette.

I have almond-shaped eyes, so I like to do a lighter color on the lid and a darker color in the crease. Daytime colors are matte cream, tans, and mocha. Nighttime colors are deep plums and charcoals, with more shimmer. You'd be amazed how the right eye contour for your eye shape can completely change the look of the makeup you already own, and it only takes a minute to do!

you're using a pencil, you have to pull your eyelid to the side and press hard, which you want to avoid since it pulls on the sensitive eyelid skin. Go for the creamy, chunkier pencils, as they are much easier to apply without pulling, although creamy formulas never last as long as a thinner matte pencil or liquid liner.

Mascara

As I've gotten older, I've noticed that my lashes aren't quite as lush as they used to be. I don't want to use Latisse, which is a prescription-only drug that can make your lashes longer, because it needs to be applied every day or it stops working. I don't want to put anything near my eyes that's so powerful, and it can also change the color of your irises. Too scary for me! I do like RevitaLash, which is a lash conditioner that you paint on every night like an eyeliner. It seems to help without the side effects of Latisse, and you can easily find it online.

The best, safest way to enhance lashes is with mascara. Some of my friends swear by Maybelline Great Lash; others go for Lancôme or Dior. My choice is Chanel waterproof mascara. Also try Urban Decay's Subversion Lash Primer, a white coat that goes on before mascara and thickens lashes and makes your mascara last longer.

Be careful when applying. Do your lower lashes first, and let each coat dry thoroughly so you don't get those dreaded little dots. Do all your eye makeup first so there aren't any flakes of color on the rest of your skin!

Don't Toss Your Unused Makeup—Have a Party Instead!

Yes, everyone has The Drawer or The Shelf. You know, the ones full of those skincare or makeup impulse buys that looked so glam when you bought them but you never used. My grandmother always said "waste not, want not," so here's what I do with my, *ahem*, bad choices: I have a makeup party. I invite my friends over and tell them to bring their unwanted items. They can wipe their old lipsticks with an alcohol-saturated cotton pad, but ditch the mascara and liquid eyeliner, as they can't be shared for fear of eye infections. As soon as my friends arrive I pour the champagne, and then we get down to the important business of trading. It's a win/win for everyone.

Fake Eyelashes

I prefer lashes that are short, dark, and natural looking. I realize "natural-looking fake lashes" is an oxymoron, but I don't want to look like a cartoon. I wear fake eyelashes when I work on a set or make a red-carpet appearance. They're great for bumping up your natural lashes, and you might be surprised how easy they are to apply. (I don't like the way lash extensions look—they're too long and remind me of Mr. Snuffleupagus, my *Sesame Street* childhood friend!) Duo makes a nice glue that's gentle enough to wear every day; they have a latex-free version which is especially good for me, as I have a latex allergy.

If you take off the lashes carefully, you can wear them more than once. Don't ever "rip" them off—even if you're exhausted and have had too much champagne. (I've *heard* this can happen—ha!) When you do that you are basically waxing your eyelashes—not good! You can get bald spots this way, and lashes take forever to grow back. Use a gentle eye makeup remover, soak a cotton pad, and remove gently.

Eyebrows

Don't neglect your brows! Using a brow pencil or powder will give you a polished, professional-looking face even if you aren't wearing a stitch of makeup otherwise. It's the single easiest thing you can do to make your face look youthful.

I recommend going to an eyebrow *specialist*. I go crazy when I see someone at the nail salon with their brows getting waxed by one of the nail technicians. You need a trained expert, because once your brows are properly shaped, you can take care of the strays yourself—it's like coloring in the line.

It's very important to have an eyebrow pencil or powder with a slanted brush to fill them in. My preferred brand is by Trish McEvoy. They make what looks like a mechanical pencil, in the color Natural Brunette, and doing my brows couldn't be easier.

Because my brows have been well shaped by a professional, I take care of them myself. My tweezers have my name engraved on them, basically. (Just kidding, but they could!) I much prefer tweezing to waxing or threading. Get a good, lighted magnifying mirror and it's super quick to yank out those strays! (Then turn it off because those 10x mirrors are my idea of hell once you start examining your skin!)

If you color your hair, discuss eyebrow color with your colorist before you begin. If you are not "on trend" with the color, you will look dated and,

---

Stephanie Tip: For brow color: If you're blonde to light brown, use light brown to medium brown; if you're medium to dark brown, match the color; for black hair, mix black and dark brown; for grey, a nice taupe is appropriate. If you want more of a natural brow, use a powder and do not start at the beginning of the brow. This is a huge mistake because most of the color on the brush will be deposited at the beginning of the brow, making it look too harsh. Start just before the center of the brow, follow through until the end, and then go back to the beginning and do that last.

---

therefore, old. Don't go too dark or you'll end up looking like Ernie's pal, Bert!

It's also important to trim your brows; like the hair on your head, it can get overgrown. Use nail scissors, or ask your hairstylist to do it. Barbers always do it for their male clients!

One last tip: Don't *ever* drink and pluck. If you do, things will go very badly!

Makeup for Your Lips

Lipstick and Lip Liner

If there's one item in my makeup bag I could never live without, it's my Wet *n* Wild Lip Liner in Brandywine #666. (The truth is the devil's in the details, and this detail is *amazing*!) A makeup artist put me on to it years ago and I'm so glad she did. It's a universally fabulous natural lip color, a sort of beige-rose, that works on every skin tone.

A lip liner is essential for anyone worried about those little lines around their lips. Liners keep any lip color from bleeding into your skin. It won't come off when you eat and it won't change color. It also shapes and defines your lips.

What I do is easy: I line my lips with my beloved Wet *n* Wild #666 and lightly color them in. Then I put a gloss on top—usually by Chanel, as I like their consistency—and I'm good to go. In fact, I won't wear a stitch of makeup, but I've still got clear gloss on. I can't stand the feeling of drying-out lips, and my Chanel gloss is like a nice, shiny lip balm that keeps my lips hydrated. It's not sticky like a lot of other brands that make you feel like you've got gloppy candy on your mouth.

If I wear lipstick, I like putting a dab of gloss in the middle of my top and bottom lips to make them look fuller. Or, if you're doing the matte lip look, you can use a light shimmer like you might use for your eye shadow and dab that in the middle of your upper and lower lip. It will give you the same effect.

Stephanie Tip: Use makeup as one of the tools in your skincare arsenal. It's not just something that's fun or extravagant; it can enhance however you're feeling about yourself and your tasks for the day. Having that tiny bit of color on your face can make you feel so much better!

I'm not a lipstick hoarder like a lot of my friends, most of whom still only wear one or two colors. I advise them to lighten their palette, as this looks fresher and they look younger. Rethink your palette if you change your hair color, too. Ask your colorist for advice—believe me, they know color!

Most of all, have fun with your lips. A new lipstick might be a cheap thrill, but it's so easy to change your look with a few swipes of a brilliant color. Remember, though, that just because a color is "hot" doesn't mean it will work on you! There was a color out a few years ago that made me look like I had been in the pool too long. Yuck! Try on the trendy color, go do some shopping, then reconsider. As with foundation, lighting can have a dramatic effect on lipstick colors, too.

◇◇◇◇◇◇◇◇◇◇◇◇◇◇◇◇◇◇◇

There's so much we can do to disguise, enhance, and create with a swipe of a brush that we shouldn't negate its power. Plastic surgery can be staved off for many more years with proper skincare and makeup techniques.

Next up is hair . . . let's not forget the story of Samson, whose haircut robbed him of his power, or *Tangled*, when magical long blonde hair lost its power when it was cut short and turned brunette. *Blasphemy!* Read on to learn how to wield your power effectively and fabulously!

CHAPTER
2

Heather's Hollywood Anti-Aging Haircare How-To

Hair is important. We classify whole days by how it looks, as in "I'm having a bad hair day," and everyone totally understands. Your hair is the first thing people see and judge you on when you walk into a room. A great haircut and color will *always* make you seem youthful, so use this chapter to help you take care of it and find the best looks—and use some of the tricks you'll read about to make it seem as vibrant as you feel!

We have a saying in my house: *It's just hair.* You can cut it and dye it and do all sorts of things to it. It will *always* grow back!

I had a lot of hair when I was little, and my mother decided that because I had a short forehead and a widow's peak, bangs were the best option. Once I hit those preteen years in the 1980s and started paying more attention to my hair, waterfall bangs were all the rage. I kept them in place with enough hairspray to poke a hole in the ozone layer. If you're my age, do you remember the fabled Aussie Sprunch Spray? They should have called it crunch spray, because at the end of the day your hair was dry and shellacked, like each strand had been glued, and if you laid down, it felt like your hair was going to break. It smelled like grapes and was *fabulous*!!!

Once I moved to Los Angeles, I quickly realized that there was a particular look for the young actresses in town. We wanted to look neutral so we could play a variety of roles, and we knew we had to be classic and sexy without being too specific or different. I wasn't yet familiar with flat irons, so my long, beautiful mane ended up being pretty frizzy sometimes. There is an episode of *Married with Children* that still runs, and when you see me in it, my hair is enormous! So, it was all about long, straight, pretty hair. (Let's be honest: this is Los Angeles, so make that long, straight, pretty *blonde* hair! Aside from the wig I wore while singing as Miss Lilly in the Golden Horseshoe Jamboree show at Disneyland, I was *not* going to be a blonde. Being a brunette New Yorker in Hollywood was a novelty at the time, so it really helped me stand out.)

Once I started working regularly, I could experiment a bit. I encourage everyone to have fun and play around with their hair. I've had many different lengths and styles. Terry wasn't crazy about the shaggy, chopped-up, shorter length I sported on NBC's *Stark Raving Mad*; he called it my "sitcom look." I enjoyed mixing it up, though. The key is to have a style that you can re-create. What's the point of having it look fabulous for one day out of the salon and then terrible because you can't replicate what they did? I even took my son to the salon to teach him how to make his naturally thick, coarse hair get spiky. And just so you know, reality TV doesn't provide hair and makeup artists since it's your "reality," so it's necessary to know how to do your hair.

Because hair is so important, it can change our image and the way we feel about ourselves. That's why when we go through a breakup, we often go to our hairdresser because we need a fresh start. Hair can also be used as a decoy. Had a nose job? Get a dramatic new hairstyle or color and people think *that's* what's different about you. Do you remember that ABC after-school special series? I used to watch every week. One in particular was about a girl who used a new hairstyle as a decoy so people wouldn't notice her new mouth full of braces! I once read that Gwyneth Paltrow doesn't feel dressed unless her hair is blown out and straight. Even stunning Gwyneth feels more confident with great hair.

Remember how thick and full and easy to care for your hair was when you were a teenager? I do, and I sure miss that hair! As we age and our hormone levels start to decline, our hair changes along with our skin and nails and teeth. It thins. It loses moisture and gets drier more quickly. Its luster disappears. Worse, it loses its color and starts to go grey or white.

So how do you get sensational hair that makes you look and feel youthful? The last thing you want to have is a hairstyle that makes you look older than you are, that isn't quite right for your face shape, or that's tired and drab. Not when there are so many incredible options to help you have the hair of your dreams.

These are my favorite hair tips, along with those from my Hollywood hairstylist, Kelly Kline:

1. Feed your hair like you feed your body!

I always believed that you are what you eat and that as long as you eat healthy, then you're getting all the nutrients you need for beautiful hair, skin, and nails. That's just not the case. As it turns out, me, who had *never* taken a supplement, *ever*, was shocked to learn that I needed one once my hair started to show visible signs of aging. This is why Terry and I created our Beaute Caps, which contain hyaluronic acid, collagen, amino acids, vitamins, other beauty super-foods, and, most importantly for hair (as well as nails and skin), eight thousand micrograms of biotin.

Biotin is a water-soluble B vitamin, so if you ingest more of it than is needed, you excrete it in your urine. It's needed for proper cell metabolism and to transport carbon dioxide away from your cells. Researchers aren't quite sure of the exact mechanism behind biotin's efficacy, but it is likely due to its effect on keratin, the basic protein component of hair, nails, and skin.

I've gotten so many Instagram messages and calls from chemo patients telling me that our Beaute Caps have revitalized their hair. I saw how my own hair went from thin to much thicker, and it seemed to grow faster, too. My nails are also a lot stronger. So I recommend a good supplement with biotin in it (although, of course, you must discuss all your supplementation with your physician, especially if you have any underlying health conditions).

Also, one of the best things you can do for your hair is a scalp massage. Getting that blood flow going helps stimulate your hair follicles. I'd rather have a short scalp massage than a long body massage!

2. Discussing your hair with your stylist is as important as getting the cut.

Like a great makeup artist, a great hairstylist can completely transform your appearance. Nothing rocks my world more than seeing one of my friends walk into the room with a head-turning new do! After years of ultra-luxe long, blonde locks (augmented with extensions), one of my best friends decided she needed a change. Without even a mention (and we talk about *everything*!), she ditched the extensions and cut her hair into a "lob," the trendy term for a super-chic long bob. Absolutely stunning. Even though her husband isn't crazy about it, everyone else thought she looked straight off the runway! (Why do men only seem to like long, straight hair? Terry's opinion is that men want to look in a woman's face rather than see hair go all over the place!) She said she tried it because she trusted her hairdresser, and he thought this would look great on her. He was right.

A bad haircut, on the other hand, can not only make you cry but can age you overnight, so it's crucial for you to go to your stylist with a lot of ideas. Don't use words—bring photos from fashion or hair magazines, or pull up images from different websites. It makes your stylist's job so much easier when you are candid. They want you to be happy, and you want to have your looks enhanced, not dominated or diminished, by your haircut.

As with makeup colors, you should also be realistic about how the latest trends are going to look on you. If you have a very angular face, for example, a severe bob might not be the best idea. If you hate the feel of hair on your face like I do, bangs could be an issue. If you like the versatility of shoulder-length hair, you need to think about how you're going to feel after you take the plunge and ask for a super-short cut—it could be as liberating for you as I found mine, or you could hate it!

You know who you are inside and what you want to be outside. A great stylist will ask a lot of questions in order to get a good idea of your personality, likes, and dislikes, and will then be able to figure out what will suit your facial structure and build. But that doesn't mean they have the last word. If you really want to do something, do it! If you're scared about making drastic changes, then do it incrementally. Remember: *It's just hair.* It grows back.

3. Factor your lifestyle into your hairstyle.

My battle with bangs continued, and every time I cut them I love them for two days but then I go, "*Why* did I do that?" I have a cowlick in the front of my hair so if I have to plaster my bangs down in any kind of humidity it's a disaster.

I definitely need to listen to my own advice! Your lifestyle is an important component of your discussions with your hairstylist. If you work out every day and take a lot of showers, or are very, very busy and don't have time for hairstyling that necessitates a blow-dryer, you need a low-maintenance cut, especially a short one that falls into place, or one that you can pull back into that all-purpose ponytail. If you like to play around with different styles, you need a length that gives you versatility. If you work in a corporate environment with a dress code (you have all my sympathy if you do!), going for something super avant-garde won't be on your radar.

4. Don't get stuck in a hair rut—it's guaranteed to make you look older.

Although I have a go-to look for my makeup, I still like to experiment and try to change it up. Ditto with my hair. I know that my hair looks best as it is now, and that being a brunette suits me best, but I'm trying new looks. You might not see me out in public with them, but I'm sure having fun in the privacy of my bathroom! And why not? It's just hair! You won't know how a style looks until you try it.

If you're wearing it in the same style that you wore in your high-school yearbook photo, we need to talk. I mean, you aren't wearing the same clothes as you did in high school or college, right? (Please, *please* tell me you aren't, unless it's some insane vintage couture piece of fabulousness your mother gave you and you wear it sparingly!) If so, your hair rut is guaranteed to make you look older than you are.

Some women make the mistake of thinking that long, long hair is going to make them look younger, but that's a bit silly, especially if it's not trimmed properly; long hair (or any length hair, for that matter) with fried dead ends isn't sexy. On the other hand, short hair can be aging, too, if it's not cut in a modern style. Beauty shop–looking hair that's short and curled with volume—you know, the kind our moms went to get every week as they sat with rollers under the hot dryer—really doesn't look youthful on anyone. Sometimes a little bob can make your face rounder, which is a more youthful look if you have an angular face. Sometimes if you have a round face and you cut it too short so that the hair hits your cheekbones in just the wrong place, it can make you look heavier than you are.

What else ages you? Hair that is blown out or flat-ironed to be super straight, or hair that is blown out with too much volume. The idea is, unless you are in a theatrical production or going out for a black tie evening, your hair should look naturally and effortlessly gorgeous. Teasing and spraying your hair in a bouffant style is too dated. Flat-ironing your hair within an inch of its life makes it look thin and flat and will get stringy faster.

What *won't* age you is a style that enhances your facial structure.

Kelly Tip: People used to say that when you got to a certain age, you had to cut your hair, but not anymore. If your hair is long, I'm a huge fan of the ponytail as long as it's sleek and chic. Or, no matter what your age or face shape, you can never go wrong with a bob. Basically the length of the bob has to go with the shape of your face; you're trying to create an oval. With a round face, a bang is always good. If you have a long face, a bang is good with a bob that finishes right below your chin, shortening your face to make it look wider. If you have square face, bring it up a little shorter, right below your chin, and keep the front long so it cuts the corners off of your face. But never cut your hair when you're stressed. Emotional haircuts never work out!

You know what else ages you? I know I sound like a broken record—but it's not having fun with your hair. I know a woman of a certain age in New York City who's got the most gorgeous hair I've ever seen. It's short, and it's dyed an amazing shade of silvery lilac. It always makes me smile because she wears it with such confidence. Would I ever do that to my hair? If I thought it suited me, sure. Can I imagine my mother, who's about the same age as this woman, doing it? *Never!* It would be way too "out there" for her, but I just love this woman's attitude.

I know that everyone has their beauty line they won't cross. Some people don't want to get plastic surgery, but they'll dye their hair a dozen different colors. Some won't dye their hair, but they'll get Botox and fillers. All I'm suggesting is that playing around with hair shouldn't be thought of as a chore. Go to a hair supply store with a friend and try on some wigs. Have a laugh. You might surprise yourself by finding something that will be wonderfully transformative. Being happy with your hair will automatically make you look younger!

5. Protect your hair from the sun.

Your scalp is made up of the same skin as your face, but do you give it the same kind of protection from the sun? Yes, hair sort of works as a shield, but your parts can get painfully burned just as the rest of you can.

Sun damage, especially burns, can damage your hair follicles, and a super-dried-out scalp is not going to promote hair growth, either. Your scalp is like soil—if it's dry and cracked, it's hard for things to grow. You need a moist, rich environment, full of nutrients, to encourage the kind of growth you want. Luckily, there are sun protection sprays available at drugstores that provide an SPF as well as hydration for your hair. Always use one when you're going outside!

6. Hormones affect your hair.

My first pregnancy was especially thrilling because I didn't know what to expect. I was so excited to feel my twin babies growing, and one of the best, unexpected benefits was seeing my already thick hair become incredibly lush and even thicker thanks to those pregnancy hormones.

But as soon as those babies came out, so did my hair. In big, huge clumps.

I called Kelly, hysterically crying, and told him I was getting male-pattern baldness, and he told me that wasn't possible. I begged him to come over, and he arrived that afternoon, took one look at the balding spots on both sides of my head, and said, "Oh my God, Heather! You have male-pattern baldness!" We were freaking out, and he cut some bangs to cover the bald areas, but that didn't make me feel much better. It *wasn't* male-pattern baldness, just post-pregnancy hormones, and there wasn't anything I could do about it. My hair gradually grew back and after my fourth child it finally settled down, but it was never again as thick as it once was.

Kelly Tip: One of the best tricks for aging, thinning hair, especially if you have any balding spots, is to use a product called Toppik, which is, literally, powdered hair. It's made of keratin fibers and comes in different colors in an atomizer-like pump, and I spray it on everybody, especially when I'm working on TV shows. It sticks to your hair and instantly makes it look fuller.

You should always be paying attention to your hormone levels, especially as you get older and hit perimenopause. Declining levels of estrogen and progesterone will not only leave your skin dry, but it can cause hair loss and thinning. Changes to your hair are inevitable with age, but still, discuss any changes with your gynecologist, especially if they're sudden, and see if a short course of hormone replacement therapy might be an option. Biotin supplements should help, and a terrific cut will be able to minimize thinning spots, too.

7. Quick fixes can undo the damage.

One thing I've learned after all my years in Hollywood is that most actors don't *just* have their own hair. After years of constant styling and color changes and cuts and processing, and after spending hours on overheated sets under blazing lights, once-glorious hair can be a limp shadow of its former self. Therefore, practically every performer I know wears some kind of hairpiece, from a few extensions and clip-on bangs to full heads of weaves and wigs. They aren't embarrassed by it at all. For them, it's a professional necessity.

This is another way you can have fun with your hair. I learned this the hard way when Kelly cut my bangs one year, the morning of the *House-wives* reunion—will I *ever* learn about my bangs?—and I loved it for a day and then I hated it and had to grow them out. I should have stopped myself, as usual, and used clip-on bangs instead. (In the same realm of don't drink and pluck, do not let anyone related to you cut your bangs. Cutting bangs is actually really tricky, and if you botch it, you may well be sorry. Leave it to the pros, please!)

Kelly Tip: My favorite Hollywood trick is skin weft. It's a piece of three-inch tape with hair attached to it. You pull the strip off, part the hair, cut the strip to the size you want, stick it on, and comb your hair right over it. People will touch your head and have no idea it's there! The tape is removable with alcohol and can only be used a few times, but skin weft is much less visible than clip-on extensions and a lot of fun to play around with for special occasions.

Still, I love extensions for thinning hair. Synthetic hair is fun and affordable, but if you can afford it, try to use real hair; the quality is better. Try to match the texture of the extension to your hair, so it looks as natural as possible. Don't go too much longer, because if your hair is short and your extensions too long, you're not fooling anybody! Be very careful with how they're applied. If not, they pull your hair out by the roots when you're taking them out, and then you've created a bigger problem with broken hair and bald spots.

Clip-on extensions are genius. I use them on everyone. But here's the catch—the color isn't going to match yours and they'll look really fake, so I always color them and you should, too. Get extensions made from real human hair and ask your colorist to dye them. It's not something you can do at home. Most extension hair comes from China, so it's bleached out and then re-dyed in different colors—but to keep costs down, they use vegetable dyes that will react with the kind of color you'd be using. Not a good look!

To Dye or Not To Dye—Hair Color for the Ages

The day before my first day as a high-school senior, my mom took me to a very posh hair salon in New York City for a new haircut. She went shopping and they suggested a special kind of cut with bangs and pieces angled to layer into your face. It sounded chic and I said okay.

And then they said, "We want to lighten your tips. How does that sound?" It sounded fine, but I had *no* idea what I was getting into. About five hours and several trillion dollars later, the front of my head was like a bizarre whitish-yellow blonde and the rest of it was dark. It was so ugly and weird and I thought my mother was going to kill me, even though it hadn't been my fault! So Mom went to the drugstore and bought a box of Nice'n Easy, and we put it on that night, but the color wasn't dark enough and the bleached-out blonde bits turned a weird shade of red. I was in tears, telling my mother that I couldn't possibly go to school like that, but clearly I didn't have any choice. So, a week or so later she got another box of dye, except this time it was too dark, and all my hair came out black as a raven's. She hated it, but I thought I looked like Joan Jett. (Well, it was the '80s!) Every time I washed it, a bit of the black came out and my hair turned a different shade. What a disaster. By the end of the year, the only way to salvage it was to chop it all off.

A good colorist should prevent any hair disasters and ease you out of your comfort zone. A different shade, even one that's subtly close to your natural color, can make you look sensational and so much younger. If you want to try a new color, go for temporary or semipermanent first, as they wash out. If your hair is dark, though, you will have to get it bleached in order for the new color to be true, and this is a process that should always be done in a salon. It is tough on your hair, but a pro can minimize the damage.

I don't color my hair now, but I am starting to get grey. The first time I found one of those hairs, I freaked. Then I decided it looked blonde. I decided it was like blonde highlights. Only not blonde. *Grey!* Ugh! It's one of those moments, isn't it? Tangible proof, no matter how quickly you yank it out, that you *are* getting older! Although I realize it's ridiculous—hair-color loss is genetic—I couldn't help feeling a bit sad. Also, on a practical level, I'm a busy, working mom of four kids and the idea of sitting in a salon to color my hair every four to six weeks gave me anxiety!

Most hair colorists say that you should go lighter as you get older. That doesn't mean a dark brunette like me should go blonde, but that I could add a few highlights, or make subtle changes. Whatever you decide to do, make sure your roots don't show. Nothing, and I mean, *nothing*, is more aging than seeing an inch or more of visibly grey roots.

Factor your lifestyle into any color changes, too. If you are going grey and your roots will show quickly, you're going to need touch-ups after only a few weeks, and this is not only expensive but time-consuming and can damage your hair. You can get root touch-up products like Tween Time or Kelly's favorite, Rita Hazan Root Concealer, in drugstores, and they can help a lot and cause far less damage to your hair.

You'll also find that hair color changes your hair texture, usually for the better, because it gets a bit thicker. This makes it easier to style, but it also makes your hair more porous and it will take longer to dry.

Kelly Tip: One of the worst things you can do is color your hair at home. You're putting layer upon layer of color over it, which is why hair can turn all these weird colors and get fried on the ends. Let the pros do it! Add regular trims, which can help thinning hair look thicker, and you're going to have fantastic hair.

When the first grey hairs arrive, start with really gentle highlighting or low lights with a few foils, and that's all you need to weave in some dark. It can even be a different color to cover the greys. Have some fun! The biggest mistake is trying to make your hair the color it used to be; your youthful color is not necessarily what looks good on you now. It's much better to go two shades lighter than your natural color, as that will make you appear much more youthful. A nice, light brown color with some highlights softens your face and makes you look softer, prettier, and younger!

Heather's Haircare

Where to start with haircare products? The first thing you should do is discuss your hair texture and its condition with your hairstylist, because they are experts and can guide you to the best choices.

Depending on your hair's condition, use different products for different needs, and switch them up every few weeks. For example, if your hair is dry and colored, use volume-enhancing products one day and color boosters the next time. Most haircare products are not expensive—there is no special ingredient that warrants an outrageous price, especially as you wash them out! Save your money for makeup items that are going to stay on your skin all day!

Shampoo

Less is more with shampoos, too. I wash my hair every day, but since it's not colored, I like a basic shampoo that does a deep cleansing. Brands I prefer are Kérastase, Fekkai, Neutrogena, and Aveda. It's important to read the front of the bottle and only use one that's right for your needs: dry, damaged, colored, etc.

Conditioner and Masks

If your hair starts to look greasy near your scalp, it might be because you're using too much conditioner. It's meant to be used on the ends. Really! Only once a week (mostly on ponytail days) do I put conditioner all over my head and rub it in my scalp as a deep conditioner.

If your hair is very dry, use a dollop of conditioner on your scalp after you shampoo it, and then rinse it out. If I have time, I will do a conditioning mask every two weeks; hair masks are intensely hydrating and can

---

Kelly Tip: There's a difference between conditioning and moisturizing your hair. If you put too much conditioner on hair, it becomes brittle. A moisturizer, or a cream rinse, is designed to put moisture back in your hair and coat it to make it feel good. You need a balance of both.

---

help keep the frizzies at bay. If you like to take baths instead of showers, apply a hair mask and then wrap your head in a towel—the heat from the bath will activate it and make it more effective.

Hair Serums

Similar to serums for your skin that are loaded with potent ingredients, hair serums can be intensely nourishing for your hair and scalp. One of my favorite anti-aging products is a hair serum called Grow Gorgeous Hair Density Serum. It's practically miraculous and makes your hair feel wonderful, fuller, and even like it grows more quickly. (You can find it at many drugstores or online.) I like to apply it in the morning; I rub it into my scalp as soon as I get up, put my hair into a ponytail, add my headband, and hit the gym. The heat from my sweating during my workout helps activate the serum; after I wash my hair it looks incredible. In fact, if I could recommend only one hair product, this would be it!

Heather's Hairstyling Tips

When you're a performer, your hair is going to pay the price. Heat is really hard on your hair, and having it pulled and twisted into all sorts of styles is hard on it, too. So when I'm not working, I try to style it as little as possible. I'll just blow-dry the front and pull it all back into a bun or a ponytail because it's so easy and minimizes pulling.

When I get my hair styled, I tell the stylist *not* to use any products. This makes me probably the only woman in Hollywood to do so! But my hair gets so greasy so quickly that I literally can't put anything on it other than a bit of hair spray.

Your own hair texture is going to dictate which products will work for you. I'm sure you already know what kind yours is, and you buy products specifically for that texture or condition. The biggest mistake is to use far too much product, which will weigh your hair down.

Every product has a very specific use, so use them properly and they'll not only work better but be more economical, too. For example, you can

Kelly Tip: The most important product is a root lift. It works on all hair. My favorite is Paul Mitchell Extra-Body Daily Boost. You spray it on roots after you wash your hair, comb it through around the front and the crown, then blow-dry your hair upside down and pull straight down. Direct your hair the way you want it to go. You have a very short time to get it right. A root lift product has alcohol in it so if you dry it in the wrong direction, you have to start over again.

For hair spray, my first choice is Oribe Superfine Strong Hair Spray for use with a hot tool and Oribe Dry Texturizing Spray for a messy, beachy style. It gives hair volume and works with any kind of hair texture.

Also for styling, I love Kiehl's Creme with Silk Groom. Put it on your hands and run it through the ends to tame them. I also love R+Co Jackpot Styling Crème. It's in between a cream and a gel, and is great for spikey pixie hair-cuts or for a tousled, scruffy look.

Aside from root lift, don't put styling products on your roots. Just squirt a little bit on your fingers and rub your fingers together until it kind of disappears and apply from the ends up.

use a volumizing mousse on your roots to pump them up, and a gel or spray on the sides or ends to keep them in place.

The Tools You Need

You only need a few tools in your hair arsenal:

1. The best quality brush you can afford. Natural bristles only, please! I use a Mason Pearson brush with boar's hair bristles. Metal bristles are damaging to your hair.
2. A durable comb. One with wide teeth is ideal for wet hair, and a good rat-tail comb is ideal for making precise parts.
3. Cushy elastic bands. Never, ever use regular rubber bands, as they pull, tangle, and shred your hair!
4. A good blow-dryer. Use the lowest heat settings so you don't fry your hair!

My Two Favorite Styling Products

My favorite styling aid isn't something you spray into your hair. It's a genius invention called a Wrapadoo. It's a super-absorbent turban that you put on as soon as you're out of the shower, and it removes most of the moisture from wet hair so it takes far less time to dry. This means you can minimize your sessions with your blow-dryer—and as you know, heat is the enemy of healthy hair, and the less you need, the better the condition of your hair.

Other than that, all I use is Elnett, the most long-lasting and amazing hair spray in the world. It doesn't get sticky, it doesn't crack, it doesn't flake, and it lasts and lasts.

5. Optional: A flat iron. This is a versatile tool to smooth and straighten hair if that's the look you want. Just don't overdo it, as the heat can sizzle your hair to a crisp, and if your hair is too smooth it looks fake and can be aging. Look for a flat iron that is ceramic—it's much less damaging to your hair than a metal plate.

6. Optional: A curling iron. I love my Sarah Potempa Beachwaver. Sometimes it's nice to put a little wave in your hair, and this device makes it super easy.

Kelly Tip: If you use a good product like a root lifter, you will never need to use high settings on your blow-dryer; the cool setting will still give your roots the volume you want.

◇◇◇◇◇◇◇◇◇◇◇◇◇◇◇◇◇◇

Hope you're having fun with us so far, and gleaning a few pearls along the way . . . stay tuned because up next will be everything essential about ingredients, products, treatments, and procedures for your skin! Which, in my opinion, is a woman's *best* asset. (Along with hair and breasts!)

Products, Treatments, and
Procedures Guide

CHAPTER
3

You're Putting That on Your Skin? Smart Ingredients/ Smarter Consumers

There's nothing new about wanting to have great skin.

The ancient Greeks mixed crocodile dung with mud for their facials. Cleopatra loved to bathe in a tub full of milk and honey. The recipe for one medieval concoction contained hedgehog ashes, bat blood, bees' wings, mercury, and slug slime. Once Queen Elizabeth I painted her face white to hide her smallpox scars, the vogue for dead-white skin took off like crazy—crazy being the operative word, as the face paint was made from highly toxic white lead mixed with chalk. And to take all this dreadful stuff off their faces, women used a revolting mixture of wine and urine. Things hadn't improved much in the nineteenth century, when many people drank Fowler's solution to improve their complexions. The main ingredient? Diluted arsenic. Aren't you glad you live in the twenty-first century?

We are, but progress has its own set of problems. There are so many skincare products available that it's almost paralyzing to know what to choose. My preteen daughter and I were at a beauty superstore the other day and the choices were overwhelming for both of us! We asked four different sales associates for opinions on new products, and we got four different answers. *Ugh!* Many of the products are wonderful, of course, but beauty companies know that women looking for hope in a jar are vulnerable to exaggerated or bogus claims and can be easily seduced by the sumptuous packaging and luxurious feel of a product that, in reality, is not much different than a much cheaper drugstore brand.

So how can you make the most informed choices? Use this checklist Terry and I compiled:

1. Don't buy into the hype.

Women's magazines and blogs are full of features about the latest and greatest, along with copious ads sporting flawless models and bald-faced claims. To which we have two things to say: Photoshop, and BS!

Photoshopping and airbrushing have become so out of control in all media that it's almost impossible to know what's real or not. I used to be under the magazines' spell until I was on *Jenny*, an NBC sitcom with Jenny McCarthy in the 1990s. Jenny was the "It" girl at the time and graced the covers of many magazines. She was also the first person I ever heard of to be vocal in the media about Photoshopping. She showed me how the magazines airbrushed her skin, elongated her legs, and did all kinds of tricks—and she was *gorgeous*, with a perfect body! What would they do with the rest of us? Even teenaged models with blemish-free, beautiful skin are tweaked to remove miniscule "imperfections." Other actresses whose faces are well known to you over the years—and who, naturally, have smile lines and wrinkles and freckles—appear to be shockingly smooth-skinned. Do you think they really only use the products they're touting? *Please!*

So where does that leave us? Back at square one.

Since it's virtually impossible to see the unretouched, original advertising photos, consumers often don't realize that editorial content can sound completely accurate and doctor-vetted about the next new thing because the next new thing's manufacturer bought a lot of ads and expects positive coverage in return. Trust us—if something sounds too good to be true, it is!

2. Always read the fine print.

When ads claim that 77 or 82 or 95 percent of those tested saw visible results, you want to believe them, right? Until you haul out your trusty magnifying glass to read the fine print at the bottom of the page. At which point you will likely see that a whopping ten or twenty-three or maybe even fifty-nine women did the testing. Are those paltry figures for real? Hell, yeah. Is that the kind of testing you want to rely on? That's not exactly what we call a valid sampling.

3. Beware of buzz words.

Whenever we look at skincare packaging and/or ads, certain buzzwords set off all kinds of warning bells. Avoid these:

- ❖ *All-natural.* What do you expect manufacturers to say, "all unnatural"? Snake venom and bubonic plague are all natural. Even Botox is all natural! All natural is no more than a smoke-screen to hide the fact that this product doesn't have anything special in it.
- ❖ *No chemicals.* Here's where a little bit of science comes in handy. Everything on this planet is made up of chemicals, especially your body. So no skincare product can *ever* be free of chemicals!
- ❖ *Allergy-tested.* This category is hard to assess. A genuine allergy is a reaction by your body's immune system to something that is usually benign—and it can be lethal. (Someone with a peanut allergy must avoid a product with peanut oil in it, for example.) Often, people think they are having an allergic reaction to a product when they're really having an *irritation* reaction. The only way to know if you're truly allergic is to have testing done under the supervision of an allergy specialist.

Heather: This is an issue that's very important to me, as I am allergic to latex and certain plastics. When I noticed a few grey hairs, Kelly told me it was time for a glaze, without dye or peroxide or ammonia, and as he massaged it into my hair, I started to react. Later that night, my entire scalp was covered in blisters and so painful I had to put on a cortisone cream. At first I thought it was the glaze, but it was the gloves! Fortunately, there are latex-free gloves, but I even have to wear wire-rimmed sunglasses because plastic sunglasses left symmetrical welts on my cheeks where they touched my face.

That's why I have to be super careful with cosmetics. What people don't realize is that some products contain binding agents made from latex or plastic, and they're not going to be listed as an ingredient. I look for products with the fewest ingredients in them as possible, and always test on my arm before applying to my face. This is very important, so let me say this again—*always* test on your arm (apply a tiny bit of the product near your elbow) if you have any sensitivities or have had any reactions in the past. This is especially true for hair color, but it should be done with *everything.* I know it's a hassle, but it's worth it to avoid any kind of bad reaction or even scarring.

The only good thing about my allergies is that we know if the products we've tested work on me without any kind of reaction, they should be safe for anyone else!

- ❖ *Preservative-free.* Preservatives are used to prevent the growth of bacteria and mold and other creepy crawlies in your products. Some are totally benign and some are problematic, but they should not be demonized because your products would quickly turn rancid and ineffective without them.
- ❖ *Removes toxins.* "Toxins" is one of those buzzwords that drives us crazy. A toxin is a poison. If you ingest a poison or put one on your skin, you're going to know about it! You *can't* sweat away or flush out alleged toxins or impurities using any special kind of ingredient or food. You have something really wonderful to use to do that for your skin—it's called *soap.* And you have two things inside your body responsible for ridding it of anything perceived as toxic—namely, your liver and gallbladder.

FDA Approval Means Safe, Not Effective!

The FDA, or Food and Drug Administration, is the government agency responsible for overseeing public health. As such, it regulates the approval of items like drugs, food additives, vaccines, medical devices, tobacco products, and cosmetics.

But here's what consumers don't understand: FDA approval only means one thing—*safe*. It doesn't mean effective, it means *safe* and will cause no harm when used as directed. A drug that is FDA-approved can still kill you, of course, if you take too much of it!

Another big problem with touting FDA approval is that the agency does not regulate herbal supplements and botanicals. Instead, herbs and botanicals (such as an essential oil) are classified as dietary supplements, so they are exempted from the more rigorous standards used by the FDA for food, drugs, and medical devices. There is absolutely no way for a consumer to know if these ingredients are safe or if they provide the dosage level they claim.

So, yes, you need to use ingredients that are FDA-approved, but that doesn't mean they're going to work.

4. Learn how to read a label.

You read the labels on food items you're thinking of buying, don't you? (Well, if you don't, you know you should!) It's just as important to know what you're putting *on* your body as it is to know what you're putting *in* it. See page 50 for details on how to read a beauty product label.

5. Use products with MD-grade ingredients.

Physicians and surgeons who sell products with their names on the label are selling their reputations as well. Hopefully, they will have access to knowledgeable cosmetic chemists and will ensure that the potency and efficacy of their products is high.

How to Read a Label

It's hard enough to decipher a food label, and beauty products push the limit of consumer understanding. You practically need to be a chemist to pronounce, much less figure out, what's listed on the box!

1. First, look for active ingredients.

There are two components to the ingredient list: "active ingredients," and everything else. You'll see active ingredients listed only if a drug is in the product. This will be highlighted in a "Drug Facts" box listing the active ingredients, the percentage of concentration, and the usage. For all other ingredients, you will not be able to tell the percentage of their concentration unless the manufacturer specifically adds that information.

If an over-the-counter (OTC) product doesn't have a Drug Facts box, it does *not* contain any ingredient that can "penetrate" down to the deepest skin layers where the real healing takes place. Only prescription drugs like Retin-A can do that. So if you see collagen listed, for example, realize that this collagen will remain on the surface of your skin; it *can't* do what the manufacturer is assuming you want it to do!

2. Next, look at the other ingredients.

Skincare ingredients are always listed in descending order of concentration. Usually, the top three are the most important, and one of them is usually aqua, or plain old water, which is needed for any cream or liquid other than an oil.

But this descending list can be a bit tricky for consumers. If the product is being touted as containing a specific (and often very costly) ingredient but it's at the very bottom of the list, you know it's there in only minute quantities. But, to be fair, some ingredients are so highly concentrated, such as fragrance, that only a tiny bit is needed—and it will be at the bottom of the list. It can be extremely difficult to know how much of an ingredient will actually be effective, and you can be sure that manufacturers are not going to tell you.

Do You Really Need Skincare Supplements?

This is a controversial topic, with conflicting studies and opinions. We believe that even when you eat the healthiest diet possible, nutrients go first to your major organs—your heart, lungs, liver, brain, and all the rest—so your skin, hair, and nails get the dregs. Makes sense, of course, to keep you alive, but this also means your skin can be paying the price. This is why we created Consult Beaute's Beaute Caps, with vitamins, minerals, amino acids, antioxidants, and, especially, biotin, which you read about in chapter 2.

Discuss this with your physician. If you decide to take a supplement, do your research and buy a reputable brand; otherwise, you could not only be wasting your money but endangering your life. The FDA does *not* regulate supplements, so there's no way to know what's in those capsules unless you get them tested, and an ordinary consumer can't do that. It's *absurd*. Random testing has found that some brands not only don't contain the potency listed, but they are made up of other ingredients altogether! This is very scary—you could be allergic and unwittingly take something that could cause a severe reaction or, at the very least, be completely ineffective. Then you get the double whammy of not only wasting your money but not seeing results and thinking the supplement is useless when you really do need it!

Ingredients to Avoid

Put these ingredients on your watch-out list:

❖ *Apricot or any pits in facial scrubs.* Because the skin on your face and neck is so tender, you never want to use scrubs with rough particles in them. They can leave your face irritated and raw. Save them for the calluses on your feet!

❖ *Formaldehyde.* A toxic carcinogenic embalming chemical, current law stipulates that cosmetics can't contain it in any quantity that would be harmful unless you're particularly sensitive to it. Still, why risk it?

❖ *Hydroquinone.* The most effective and reliable ingredient to reduce pigmentation when applied topically, hydroquinone has become a very controversial skin lightener because of concerns it may cause cancer, as it does so in rats exposed to it. It's still FDA-approved in 0.5 to 2.0 percent for OTC products and 4 to 12 percent in prescription doses. A study by the *International Journal of Toxicology* suggested that it not be used in any leave-on cosmetics and only in small concentrations in rinse-off products, but Terry believes there is no evidence it causes problems in humans; no cases have been reported. (*Aspirin* can cause problems in lab rats, too, just so you know!) It can make the skin sun-sensitive, so you must use a sunscreen with an SPF of at least 25, applied every hour or two on the treated areas, when outdoors.

❖ *Mineral oil.* This is another popular ingredient where some claim it's a fabulous hydrator and others claim it's a guaranteed pore clogger, stealing moisture from skin cells and leading to collagen and connective tissue breakdown and skin aging. I think there are better ingredients, such as calendula and chamomile extracts, coconut oil, and petrolatum, so you should avoid it.

❖ *Parabens.* Parabens are a preservative with a bad rap due to a decade-old study that found them in breast cancer tissue. There isn't any evidence to suggest that parabens caused the cancer in the first place, or that it's harmful in cosmetics, but many consumers still don't want to risk using it.

❖ *Phthalates.* Now banned in baby bottles, phthalates are used in plastics and may be an endocrine disruptor, meaning they affect your hormones. Listed as chemicals of concern by the Environmental Protection Agency (EPA), they should be avoided until they're determined to be completely safe.

❖ *Sulfates.* Sulfates are chemicals called surfactants that help products foam up, but they can strip all the oils off your hair, leaving it dry and broken. You know how foamy the cleansers are at the car wash? That's due to sulfates. They might be great for your tires but they can be hell on your hair. Although most drugstore brands contain sodium lauryl or sodium laureth sulfate, you can find good ones (often organic brands) that are labeled sulfate-free. They might not be as foamy, but they're better for your hair and scalp.

◇◇◇◇◇◇◇◇◇◇◇◇◇◇◇◇◇◇◇

Now that you know what to look for on the labels, read on for a comprehensive guide to OTC skincare products. We're going to show you what works best for the most common skincare issues.

CHAPTER
4

Over-the-Counter Skincare Products Guide

Your skin is amazing stuff. It's elastic and pliable. It lets you touch and *feel*. It keeps the elements out, and it cools you down when the heat is on. It regenerates as it heals itself and rarely gets infected. But because skin is just, well, *there*, it's easy to take it for granted. To leave it unprotected. To not replenish it. To try all sorts of crazy new products or treatments on it and then complain that it isn't responding—or, worse, giving you a rash or zits or splotches or wrinkles.

Take care of your skin and it will take care of you.

Read on, and we'll teach you about the different kinds of over-the-counter (OTC) products, available without a prescription. (*Note:* Terry and I wrote this chapter together; he did the science and I tackled the consumer angle.)

Basic Skin Function

Your skin has three different layers:

❖ *Stratum corneum.* The stratum corneum is the outermost layer. It's made up of interlocking dead skin cells that rise to the surface, pushed up there by the new, living cells underneath. This process is constant throughout your lifetime, but there's a catch. In young people, skin cell turnover takes place about every three weeks. As you get older, the process slows, and it can take up to forty-five days. That's why exfoliation is so important—it gets rid of the old, dead skin cells and allows the fresher skin underneath to appear.

❖ *Epidermis.* Just beneath the stratum corneum is the living yet thin layer called the epidermis. It contains three types of cells: keratinocytes, made up of a tough protein; melanocytes, which contain melanin, the pigment that gives your skin its color; and Langerhans cells, which aid your immune system in fighting off infections.

❖ *Dermis.* The bottommost layer of skin is the dermis. It's made up of two proteins, collagen and elastin. Collagen is comprised of cells called fibroblasts that weave themselves into bundles to provide strength and durability for your skin. Elastin filaments are what allow your skin to hold its shape. Once these filaments are stressed by external assaults like cigarette smoke, sun exposure, or pollution, as well as internal assaults like the (ugh) inevitable aging process, they start to sag. This is why skin gets droopy as you get older.

Why Does Skin Age?

Even if you take the best possible care of your skin, it's still going to visibly age. Cells die, and the previously strong and durable collagen and elastin fibers lose their oomph. At the same time, the muscles in your face become weaker and looser—and this makes them sag. Your skin gets stretched out over these sagging muscles and droops and gets wrinkles. To make things even more annoying, the fat pads in your face—what had once given you such deliciously pinchable cheeks when you were a toddler—lose volume, too.

You can't control the genetic factors that make your skin age—some people are more prone to wrinkling or drier skin than others. But you *can* control the extrinsic factors that can unwittingly add years to your appearance.

How to Clobber Your Skin

Nearly all of the factors that influence how your skin ages are habits that *you* control. Good habits (balanced diet, regular exercise, going on stress-busting mini vacations) and bad habits (ha-ha, where to get started?). How you choose to live *now*, not your genetic heritage, has the greatest impact on facial aging, which means that you can easily make a huge difference in your appearance at any age.

Most people think it's almost impossible to stop Mother Nature's reign over the ravages of sun damage (what dermatologists refer to as photoaging). Luckily, it isn't. Dermatologists used to believe that 80 percent of your skin damage was already done by age eighteen, but they were wrong. Figure that about 10 percent of damage to your skin happens every decade from external factors, such as sun exposure, meaning *you* can control 90 percent of the factors affecting how you age. Cross these behaviors off your list and you will instantly look better:

❖ *Getting fried in the sun.* We see people baking on the beaches here in California and can't believe they're out there unprotected. Go to the section on page 76 for more info on how UV radiation not only can turn you an unflattering shade of lobster, but how it accelerates the aging process. Sun exposure is the *number one cause* of premature skin aging. More sun = more wrinkles = less elasticity = more drooping = you need help!

❖ *Exposure to the elements.* I grew up in New York State when the winters were brutal. Factor in all the pollution and you can watch all the dewiness get sucked right out of you. I might not have to deal with winter anymore, but I do have to face the lower production of skin oils as I age, so I've had to switch up my moisturizer for something more protective and hydrating.

❖ *Boozing it up.* Many studies have shown that drinking a five-ounce glass of red wine with dinner every night has health benefits—the wine is loaded with antioxidants (primarily resveratrol from the grape skins and seeds) and can improve cardiovascular health and good cholesterol levels, as well as help prevent cell degeneration and, perhaps, even certain diseases. But did you know that excessive drinking will not only ruin your health, but will make you look as bad as you feel?

Overdoing the frozen margaritas is dehydrating. Too much booze stresses your liver, which is detox central in your body. It robs your body of essential nutrients. Alcohol also contains a compound called acetaldehyde, which breaks down the collagen fibers in your dermis. This is why so many alcoholics have terrible, parched, wrinkled skin.

❖ *Smoking.* Terry can always ID the smokers when they come in for a consultation, even if they lie about it (which they often do). Their skin is ashy and they have telltale lines above their lips from all that pursing while they inhale. Wonder why? According to information from the American Lung Association, the approximately six hundred ingredients in a cigarette create a whopping seven thousand chemicals when they're smoked; at least sixty-nine of them are known to be carcinogenic and many are toxic, too. As resilient as your skin is, it can't fight the onslaught of this poisonous crap—not just from when you inhale but from all the smoke wafting around your face.

❖ *A crummy diet.* Eating the wrong kind of food doesn't just make you fat; it makes you unhealthy. Scarf down a lot of white and beige foods (especially white sugar, processed flour, and packaged junk food) and your skin is going to look as bland and blah as those colors. Eat a lot of brilliantly colorful fruits and vegetables instead and you'll be getting valuable micronutrients and antioxidants, feeding your brain and body as well as your skin. The old adage "you are what you eat" holds true!

❖ *Not enough sleep.* There aren't enough hours in the day for me to do my work, see my children, take care of the household, talk to my friends, pay attention to what's going on in the world, and maybe squeeze in a few minutes with my husband. I need at least eight hours of uninterrupted sleep every night. Do I get them? *Ha!* Luckily, Terry doesn't need as much sleep as I do, which is a good thing for his patients when he spends up to twelve hours a day doing the surgical procedures he loves.

Yet chronic sleep deprivation not only wreaks havoc on your immune system; it's also hell on your skin. Just look at workers pulling double shifts. Their skin is a paler shade of grey. There's a reason it's called *beauty sleep*. It's not just a good idea, it's a *necessity*.

❖ *Stress.* Why do your friends and loved ones know when you're stressed to the max, even if you say everything's fine? Because it shows in your skin. When I get stressed, I can't sleep, I eat poorly, and I'm irritated by everyone. As for Terry, he does the same—but he's a man so he won't recognize it or admit it! (Can you hear me laughing? Well, I am! *Ha!*)

This is what we try to do about it: we work out regularly, stay out of the pantry late at night, and remember to have sex. Never negate the positive power of human connection. It makes you feel good and beautiful and younger. And it helps you get deeper, more refreshing sleep.

Conscious breathing is a great stress buster. So are stretches. So is listening to music you like. Or taking a hot, scented bath in a darkened room with the door closed and all distractions left outside. Exercise is one of the easiest and most effective ways to manage your stress. It clears your mind, improves your breathing, tones your body, strengthens your cardiovascular system, and helps you lose weight. There is no downside to it (unless you are like some people we know and never do one trendy workout if they can do fifteen—and have the injuries to show for it). Bodies need to move, so you need to find the time to add a regular exercise routine into your life. That doesn't mean you need to schlep to the gym—brisk walking is one of the best exercises you can do. So, get moving! Nothing is more youthful than the rosy glow on your face when you get the blood pumping.

Acne Care

Zits are the pits, literally! Acne scarring can certainly age us. Terry wrote the book *The Acne Cure* to help everyone not only understand this condition but to easily get rid of it for good, especially since you can develop a devastating case as an adult. That happened to me—see page 172 in chapter 8 for more.

Acne is genetic—if your parents had it bad, you probably did, too. It starts when the sebum produced by the oil glands in your skin gets clogged in your pores. This causes inflammation, and triggers the *P. acnes* bacteria on your skin to get out of control. It's exacerbated, for reasons we still don't fully understand, by hormonal fluctuations and stress.

Because seeing zits usually induces sheer panic, most people rush out to the drugstore and grab a whole bunch of products that dry out their skin and paradoxically allow more zits to form. Follow this regimen instead and your acne should disappear for good.

Meant to Do

Get rid of the zits and stop new ones from forming!

How It Works

Here is how this ingredient combination works:

1. Cleanse with a salicylic acid cleanser, no stronger than a 2 percent concentration. Salicylic acid is a fabulous anti-inflammatory and antioxidant. Be sure there are no other ingredients (especially glycolic acid) in your cleanser.

2. Use a separate glycolic acid cream or lotion, with a concentration of 8 to 10 percent and with no other active ingredients. Apply it after you wash with salicylic acid, leave on for a few minutes, then rinse off with warm water.

3. Follow with benzoyl peroxide, which is what kills the P. acnes bacteria without harming your skin. The trick is to make the benzoyl peroxide cold. This shrinks your blood vessels as it opens up your pores so it can effectively penetrate into them to kill the bacteria causing the inflammation. Keep the benzoyl peroxide in your fridge. Cool your skin first by running an ice cube over it. Apply the benzoyl peroxide where it's needed and then use a cold pack for up to ten minutes.

When You'll See Results

Follow this regimen and your acne should be cleared within six weeks, although you should see some improvement right away.

Ingredients to Look For

Salicylic acid, glycolic acid, benzoyl peroxide.

Stop Using This If

If your skin gets irritated, stop using your products immediately. Continue to ice your face and try washing with Cetaphil, a very mild cleanser. If your acne is stubborn, see a dermatologist pronto!

Anti-Aging: Dry Skin on Your Face and Body

Moisturizers, Oils, and Serums

Your skin is exposed to the elements every day, and it gets thirsty. Feed it the hydration it needs!

Meant to Do

Moisturizers for your face are not treatment creams. They have one simple function: to provide hydration. They can come in the form of creams, lotions, or oils. Look for one that's noncomedogenic, or non-pore-clogging. Serums used in conjunction with moisturizers are more concentrated, with more potent ingredients that can be a very valuable addition to your skincare arsenal. Always apply a serum first, and let it soak in. Then apply a moisturizer and/or sunscreen on top.

About Masks

Masks are concentrated treatments that can tackle a wide range of skincare issues—for hydration, to purify, to exfoliate, or to just smell luscious and make your skin feel soft and smooth. I love masks and use Consult Beaute Volumagen Re-Imaging Treatment three times a week. Once you find one you like, there's no downside, because they're so user-friendly. Just be careful not to get a mask or treatment in your hairline, or you may end up with an accidental wax when you go to remove it!

Don't ignore the rest of your body. Although your facial skin is thinner and more exposed to the elements, all skin gets dehydrated and needs daily care. Your body skin can tolerate richer products with less potential for irritation.

How It Works

When you coat your skin with a good cream, oil, or serum, it blocks moisture from evaporating and temporarily makes your skin look plumper and dewier. It should also contain a humectant, which is an ingredient that attracts moisture from the atmosphere and draws it into your skin.

When You'll See Results

If your skin is very dry, you will see results right away. Products for your body work best if you apply them to damp skin.

Ingredients to Look For

Ceramides (for dry, itchy skin), glycerin (for water absorption), hyaluronic acid (filling in fine lines and crepey skin), lactic acid (exfoliating, moisturizing), petrolatum (humectant), and urea (exfoliating, moisturizing).

Stop Using This If

You have any kind of reaction or irritation.

Anti-Aging: Loss of Firmness and Elasticity, Sagging, and Crepey Skin on Your Face

Gravity sucks! You get old; you sag. You go in the sun; you sag. Time to do something about it!

Meant to Do

Firming products are *not* wrinkle products. They are designed to work against sagging or drooping skin, and make it appear tauter.

How It Works

The two best ways to firm up skin are to increase the amount of water at the surface and to decrease the amount of collagen destruction. Ingredients deposited onto the skin that attract moisture from the deeper surfaces fill out the surface of the skin, making it look tighter and more luminescent. Ingredients that decrease collagen breakdown make the skin firmer and improve elasticity.

When You'll See Results

Right away—temporarily.

Ingredients to Look For

Dehydrated marine collagen filling spheres, hyaluronic acid filling spheres, and ceramides for moisture; alpha hydroxy acids (AHAs), retinols, and vitamin C to decrease collagen breakdown.

Stop Using This If

You don't see results. This is one category where it makes more sense to move right along to the next level—you'll save money and frustration in the long run.

Anti-Aging: Loss of Firmness and Elasticity, Sagging, and Crepey Skin on Your Neck

Dear Neck: Please forgive me. Do you have to remind me of my grandmother every time I look in the mirror? Yes, I know, I took you for granted. I forgot that you're actually thin and vulnerable. I know I didn't glop sunscreen on you like I did on my face. But did you have to start going all saggy and crepey on me? *Sheesh*. So sorry! I won't do it anymore if only you'll go back to smooth and unlined. What? You *can't*? Oh yeah? Well, thanks a bunch. Love, Heather.

At the *Real Housewives of Orange County* reunion one year, everyone was talking about how great our faces looked and how bad our necks looked. This scared the crap out of me! I started begging for the technology from Terry to tighten and dissolve the fatty pad under my chin. Trust me—it's not easy, and it's getting worse, as everyone looks *down* so much these days that we're developing Tech Neck. Like the rings on a tree—not cute!

Meant to Do
Minimize the saggy or crepey chicken skin on your neck.

How It Works
Pulling moisture and water molecules from the deeper layers and reducing collagen breakdown fill the fine lines and increase the elasticity of crepey neck skin.

When You'll See Results
Right away, as long as your expectations are low. When you find the right treatment, you should see results within twenty to thirty days. Check out my neck on social media—I have become a believer!

Ingredients to Look For
Arginine, hyaluronic acid, marine collagen, retinols, vitamin C.

Stop Using This If
You see zero results even after regular use. You'll need a treatment discussed in chapter 5.

Anti-Aging: Wrinkles on Your Face

Anti-Wrinkle Products
I have friends who've told me they saw wrinkles one morning that weren't there the night before. Of course these changes were a long time coming, but, like the first grey hairs that you pluck out while screaming at your tweezers, when the wrinkles don't go away, it's time to get serious with effective OTC products.

Meant to Do

These are treatment products designed to tackle the effects of aging—and if you're starting to age, you know exactly what I'm talking about.

How They Work

By improving skin elasticity, decreasing collagen breakdown, and improving blood flow in the dermis.

When You'll See Results

Some products can make a difference right away, depending on the condition of your skin or their active ingredients. The entire Consult Beaute line was designed to give you quick results because the active ingredients get into your pores and use your own moisture to plump out your skin—this is what helps to minimize the wrinkles.

Many if not most other wrinkle treatment creams need to be given a chance to work, for up to a month. If they're truly not working, it's time to turn to chapter 5. Seeing a skillful doctor with a wide range of effective options is often less costly than your miracle-cream-of-the-week.

Ingredients to Look For

Antioxidants should be at the top of your list. They can help to slow down or even help repair skin damage and signs of aging by fighting free radicals, which are oxygen molecules that have lost an electron—leaving them wildly unstable—and will do anything to replace it. Free radicals can be formed by exposure to the toxins in the environment, such as pollution, cigarette smoke, or sun exposure. Excess free radicals cause collagen and elastin fibers to degrade, which then cause premature aging, wrinkles, and sagging. The only way to stop this is with antioxidants. You should be using them topically with your skincare products, and you should be eating them, especially nutritious fruits and veggies. This will literally feed the free radicals the extra electron they're desperately searching for and calm the little beasts down. The best topical antioxidants are vitamin C, vitamin E in the form of tocotrienol, alpha lipoic acid, and resveratrol.

About Facials

Dawn Hawley is a licensed medical esthetician who is the facialist in Terry's office. This is her advice for getting the most out of your facial:

What can a facial do for your skin? They used to be thought of as mostly a soothing and relaxing spa treatment for relaxation. Nowadays, there are many different treatments and a wide range of products available, so it's up to you to be frank with your esthetician about what you're looking for. Most of the time patients have no idea what they need—they just know what's bothering them about their skin. It's very important to find an esthetician with medical training and hands-on experience to properly treat and educate you about your needs, and who will pay attention to your lifestyle and not push a counterproductive treatment plan (for example, someone who's an avid golfer should not be following an aggressive treatment plan that makes their skin more sensitive to the sun). The last thing you want is a botched facial!

A good facial can correct as well as diminish the appearance of the aging process. Having a facial once a month gets rid of dead skin cells and stimulates new ones with more intense exfoliation techniques, followed by deep hydration. Think of it like giving your face an express car wash followed by a lustrous polish!

Be skeptical of any esthetician who applies a mask or a serum and then turns on the steam machine before leaving the room for ten or twenty minutes. I steam for less than five minutes while a clay mask or enzyme peel is on the skin instead of a massage cream. You want skin softened but not overheated—too much steam makes skin mushy, and if it's directed at your face when a very emollient cream has been applied, it can actually cause problems like blotchiness or breakouts afterward. Also be wary if there's a lot of squeezing during your facial. This is very old school, but it can cause trauma and irritation. The extraction tool should be banned from all spas;

it's good for getting blackheads out of ears, but your esthetician should only use fingertips or Q-tips.

Facials can transform your skin. For me, esthetics is, in a way, an art form. It's like creating amazing food, but instead of feeding your body I am feeding your skin from the outside in!

Next, look for peptides. These are composed of amino acid chains that are moisture binders; they act as cell communicators to help the skin to repair itself.

Retinoids are important, but it's easy to get confused about this ingredient. Retinol is a vitamin A derivative that signals directly to the skin cell to stop aging by reducing the destruction of collagen, improving blood supply, and increasing the compactness and density of the skin layers. Retinol is a lower strength than prescription-only Retin-A.

Stop Using This If

You have any kind of reaction—irritation, rashes, itchiness.

Silk Pillowcases

Meant to Do

Prevent wrinkles as you sleep.

How It Works

Silk is a unique, natural fiber with dense fibers that keep moisture close to your skin. Sleeping on silk keeps your skin cool, and because it's hypoallergenic, it's great for sensitive skin.

When You'll See Results

Right away. No more cheek creases to greet you when you're facing a bleary morning!

Ingredients to Look For

Pure 100 percent silk.

Stop Using This If

You've washed it so many times it doesn't feel the same. Never put silk pillowcases in the dryer, as this causes the silk fibers to lose their luster sooner.

Anti-Aging: Wrinkles Around Your Eyes

Anti-Wrinkle and Puffiness Eye Products

Don't you hate waking up with eyes puffier than the Stay Puft Marshmallow Man who went trampling through Manhattan in *Ghostbusters*? I know I do!

Meant to Do

Eye creams are meant to hydrate the tender skin around your eyes without causing any irritation. Some are also designed to reduce puffiness.

How It Works

Pretty much the same as moisturizers and wrinkle products.

When You'll See Results

If your skin is very dehydrated, you'll see results right away. Otherwise, expect to see changes in a few weeks.

Ingredients to Look For

In this category, it's more about not what to look for but what to *avoid*. Many skincare products contain eye-irritating ingredients; eye products are gentler and ophthalmologist-tested to ensure they won't cause stinging, itching, or burning.

Stop Using This If

Your eyes do react in any way.

Cellulite Treatments

What do you call cellulite, except maybe lumpy, bumpy, orange-peely, cottage-cheesy, or why-me? Don't forget equal opportunity offender—because an estimated 90 percent of all women, of all shapes and sizes, have it. Does that make me feel any better? Are you kidding?

I am obsessed with cellulite. I just hate it. I've tried everything to get rid of it. And let me tell you, whoever invents a 100 percent guaranteed eradicator will be a gazillionaire.

Why are we stuck with cellulite? Because women are *supposed* to have it. *Ugh!* Cellulite is basically a fat storage mechanism so that if women become pregnant and then breast-feed, they'll have adequate fat readily available for their babies. The unfortunate honeycomb appearance is because the fat is stored in little packets in our connective tissue—what connects our muscles to our skin just below the surface. (Men can't breast-feed, so their fat storage is more uniform. They have *no* idea!)

Cellulite rears its ugly head if the bands of fibrous tissue are too tight and the fat packets get squished and compressed. The trapped fat can't go anywhere and swells up, and these swollen fat cells then clump together. Cellulite often gets worse as we age, because connective tissue naturally becomes less resilient. We still don't know why some women get it so bad while others are relatively unscathed. There's a hormonal component due to estrogen, and a genetic component, too. It's just not fair!

Meant to Do

Make the cellulite disappear.

How It Works

By causing local edema (i.e., swelling), or through increasing water content.

When You'll See Results

Cellulite treatment products that create irritation work pretty quickly—usually right after you apply them. But these results are only temporary.

Ingredients to Look For

Aminophylline, caffeine, guarana.

Stop Using This If

You aren't seeing any results.

Cleansers, Toners, and Makeup Removers

Cleansers

I started my career in the theater, where I learned how my skin would pay the price if I didn't clean it properly. Stage makeup is super thick and the lights on the stage are super hot and they bake that stuff right into your face. So I don't care how tired, how drunk, or how après-sex you are—that face has got to get cleansed!

Many women think any cleanser will do the trick, but I want you to think differently. Use your cleanser to prep your skin for your treatment products the way Terry preps a patient for surgery. So when you're looking for *the* best product to spend your money on, go for the most effective cleanser you can afford—it will make all your other products that you're using *better.*

Stay away from facial cleansers that make your skin feel tight; that means it's dry and stretched. (It's the same concept as washing your hair for that squeaky-clean feeling—which means you've stripped too much oil out of it!) We want our skin to always be hydrated; youthful-looking skin is dewy and moist and has lots of elasticity.

Meant to Do

Leave your face clean and fresh without making it dry and flaky.

How It Works

Apply cleanser to damp skin, rinse, pat your skin dry, and move on to your treatment products.

When You'll See Results

Right away!

Ingredients to Look For

If you have certain skin conditions (acne, for example), you will want a cleanser that targets it. Stay away from regular soaps, as they can be very drying; choose a soap-free liquid or creamy cleanser instead.

Stop Using This If

You get irritated or break out.

Toners

Meant to Do

Many people think toners are solely meant to be astringents targeted at those with oily skin to help dry it out. That's a mistake, as it's rare for adults to have the kind of oily skin that might have plagued them as teenagers. (If you do tend toward oiliness as you get older, take heart— it helps prevent wrinkles!) The very best toners are not about stripping away but about adding hydration.

How It Works

Astringent toners strip away facial oil. Hydrating toners help create a moisture barrier.

When You'll See Results

Fairly quickly, especially if you're using a hydrating toner.

Ingredients to Look For

Avoid astringent toners with alcohol or witch hazel. Hydrating toners usually contain antioxidants.

Stop Using This If

You have any kind of reaction or irritation, especially dryness.

Makeup Removers

Meant to Do

Makeup removers are cleansers strong enough to remove waterproof mascara or the highly pigmented colors used in eye shadows, blushes, and lipsticks.

How It Works

Makeup removers are either oily or nonoily. The oily ones break down the skin's natural sebum production and rinse them out into a milky emulsion; they're best for long-lasting or water-resistant makeup. The nonoily ones contain alpha hydroxy acids like salicylic and glycolic to unstick the debris from deep pores and skin.

My Skincare Routine

Everyone I know is insanely busy, so the last thing I want to do is waste any time on taking care of my skin when a streamlined routine is all I need. I only use our Consult Beaute products because I know they give me plump, dewy, moist skin. *That's* youthful! I posted a photo not long after our line was launched and people kept asking me why my skin was so glowy . . . was it because I wearing MAC Angel Dust Shimmer or some other product? Nope. It was plain old me! Maybe I *could* have used a bit of powder to cut the grease, but never mind. I'm happy with my skin. This is what I do:

❖ *Cleansing:* I keep a bottle of our cleanser in the shower so I never forget to use it in the morning or after I work out—you never want to use deodorant soap or body cleansers on facial skin as they are too harsh.

❖ *Moisturizing and replenishment:* I use our Volumagen serum, followed by Volumagen moisturizer to make my skin plump and youthful during the day, and our Regenerol replenishment pads, serum, and cream, which is designed to resurface your skin, at night. Or, if I'm going to the gym, I'll use the Regenerol in the morning, use Volumagen after my shower at the gym, and Regenerol again at night.

I have sensitive combination skin, and I test everything because if it works on me and doesn't make me break out, it's going to work on everyone. It was very important to create a one-size-fits-all moisturizer. Bear in mind that people with very dry skin who think they need very heavy cream to moisturize usually don't.

❖ *Eye cream:* Here's a great tip—keep it in the refrigerator. It doesn't make the cream more effective but it does help with inflammation, as the cold helps reduce puffiness. That's one of the reasons why cucumbers are often recommended; they don't contain some magical property, but their high water content coupled with keeping them cool makes them hydrating.

❖ **Sunscreen:** No way am I going to age my face and get a sunburn! My favorite broad-spectrum sunscreen is Anthelios by La Roche-Posay. You can buy it at drugstores, and it absorbs instantly.

When You'll See Results

Instantly. If you wake up with raccoon eyes, your makeup remover isn't effective enough—find a different brand!

Ingredients to Look For

If your skin is very oily, you should try nonoily removers first, because the oily products, although effective, can further increase the accumulation of oils and cause blackheads and whiteheads to form.

Stop Using This If

It doesn't work well or irritates your eyes.

Discoloration and Hyperpigmentation

Lighteners and Brighteners

Many people have an uneven skin tone and/or dark or white spots, especially as they get older. They can appear as blotches or as freckles and age/liver spots. This is hyperpigmentation, which sounds complicated but is actually just the clinical term for deposits of melanin, the pigment that gives your skin color. A tan is hyperpigmentation—and sun exposure is one of the biggest reasons why you'll see these spots on your face, arms, and hands. They're harmless—just proof that you didn't use enough sunscreen!

Meant to Do

Lighteners and brighteners are meant to even out your skin tone and/or reduce spots.

How It Works

Exfoliants and bleaching agents brighten and lighten skin.

When You'll See Results

Patience is required! Most lightening/brightening agents take at least six weeks of regular use to see significant results. After three months, expect at least a 60 percent improvement.

Ingredients to Look For

If you want overall brightening and evening-out, look for alpha hydroxy acids like glycolic, azelaic, and salicylic, and products containing vitamin C. For age spots or freckles, look for a gentle bleaching agent like azelaic acid or kojic acid. Hydroquinone is FDA-approved for OTC use up to a 2 percent concentration; anything over 4 percent is prescription only.

Stop Using This If

It isn't working, your skin tone starts to look uneven, or there is any irritation.

Dull, Blah, Sluggish Skin

Exfoliants

As you learned already, your skin is always shedding itself, but skin cell turnover slows down as you age. Without an exfoliant, these cells will just sit on your skin, and sit and sit and sit, leaving your skin looking as stale as a day-old baguette. You need an exfoliant to do the job properly.

If that doesn't convince you, take a look at men your age. Why do they seem to age better? Because they shave—it's daily exfoliation! Some women do believe in this concept—it's actually an old Hollywood secret that, allegedly, Elizabeth Taylor used to do something called dermaplaning. Instead of a razor, a scalpel type of instrument gets the fuzz off.

Meant to Do

Revive your complexion so it's glowing, not sluggish and dull.

How It Works

Do you know how many skin cells you should naturally be sloughing off every minute? Oh, about thirty to forty thousand. Yes, every *minute*. Exfoliants in the form of a gentle scrub or peel remove them easily.

When You'll See Results

Within a week or two, especially if you haven't been exfoliating properly before.

Ingredients to Look For

Glycolic acid is fab stuff. It's an alpha hydroxy acid derived from sugar cane. It does a great job of sweeping away dead skin cells. Other good exfoliants are salicylic acid and fruit enzymes. You can buy OTC glycolic acid peels at a concentration up to 35 percent, but don't start playing around with peels or you can fry your skin crispier than a platter of *chicharrónes*—leave it to an experienced esthetician.

Stop Using This If

Your skin gets irritated and red and/or feels dry or rough, with flaky patches. Always start with a very gentle peel or super-gentle scrub a few times a week and work your way up to more regular use—but only if you really need it. If your skin looks good, there's no reason to go for something stronger.

Pore Minimizers

Enlarged pores are very common as you age, caused by an accumulation of oil and debris that plugs them up so they dilate and get larger.

Meant to Do

Minimize pores.

How It Works

Pore minimizers or blur products contain ingredients that smooth and prime your skin.

When You'll See Results

Right away, for at least a few hours. Bear in mind that wearing a lot of makeup, especially heavy foundation, can make pores look worse. You might want to try a primer, which smoothes the surface, and switch to a lightweight foundation. Or try a tinted moisturizer, which gives some coverage. A good trick is to mix a tinted moisturizer with a bit of regular moisturizer on the back of your hand before applying to your face, which will give you a more sheer yet polished look.

Ingredients to Look For

Microspheres and polymers that smooth the surface of your skin, peptides, and antioxidants.

Stop Using This If

You aren't getting any results.

Sun Damage

Wanna know Terry's all-time number one anti-aging tip? It's the cheapest and easiest treatment you can ever have: stay out of the sun!

Look, you are not a damask-scented rose. Or a maple tree. You need a very little bit of sun to make vitamin D, so please don't pull out that tiresome excuse for your bronzed-into-lizard skin. Sun exposure will *always* make you look older. Worse, continued sun exposure increases your risk of skin cancer by up to 78 percent. If that doesn't convince you, maybe a face full of wrinkles will!

Most sun damage comes from invisible ultraviolet UVA and UVB rays.

Think of UVA as *A = aging rays.* UVA rays can't burn your skin, but their long wavelength means they can penetrate deep down to the dermis, where they destroy collagen and elastin fibers. This damage is cumulative. It's what makes your skin sag and droop and get all wrinkled and loaded with brown and white spots. *Yuck.*

What's so scary about UVA rays is that they can zap through clouds, which is why you can get fried on a gloomy day, and glass, which is why they can harm you while you're driving or sitting at your desk in a sunny office. What's also scary is that because UVA exposure is cumulative, all the sun exposure in your youth will catch up to you, no matter what your skin tone. Yes, you can reverse some of the damage, but no, this is *not* an excuse to get a nice new bikini and hit the beach!

A tan is a response to sun damage, signaling your skin to produce more melanin to protect skin cells from even more damage. It *can't* somehow magically provide protection against burns or other damage, even if basking in the sunshine makes you feel good. Still, it's hard not to succumb to the California beach mythology and go for the glow even though I am a brunette New Yorker who likes her pale skin, except for a few occasions.

When I was at Syracuse University and had a short stint in the pageant world, I won the title of Miss Greater Syracuse and was heading to vie for Miss New York State with the hopes of competing in the Miss America pageant. I didn't win, but at least I was voted Miss Congeniality, so basically I was the nicest girl in New York for one year! Ha-ha!

Anyway, I realized that all the girls in the pageants had bronzed skin. It looked better onstage and in a swimsuit, so I headed to my local tanning salon. Unfortunately, all I ended up with was blotchy, gross skin and weird tan lines from the eye protection goggles. Yikes! I reached for a tub of Dermablend cream to even out my skin tone . . . and it got all over my white competition swimsuit. Total fail!

Then, when I went on my first trip for *The Real Housewives of Orange County,* I noticed that all the other girls were tanned blondes. This time I decided to forgo the tanning bed and get a professional spray tan instead. Putting aside my mortification about being mostly naked after four kids, standing in front of this twenty-two-year-old "expert" spray-tan girl, I did it. The problem was I was holding my boobs up so she could spray under them, and my hands got over-sprayed. I ended up looking like an Oompa Loompa with shiny orange hands that didn't match my body. Another total fail!

I think a lot of people get addicted to tanning, but tanning beds can cause extreme damage in a very short time. I really wish that people didn't think that tans make them look thinner, or that they're "healthy." They're *not.* They're proof that you're ruining your skin!

So that's the bad news about UVA rays. Unfortunately, UVB rays are even worse. Think of UVB as *B = burning rays.* These rays leave your skin as crispy crunchy as a fried onion ring any time you get a bad sunburn or even a medium tan. They cause surface damage to your skin *and* cause skin cancers.

Sunscreen

Meant to Do

A broad-spectrum sunscreen gives you some (but not total) protection against UVA and UVB rays.

How It Works

Sunscreens can contain chemical blockers (that absorb UV light), physical blockers (that reflect UV back), or a combination of both. SPF stands for Sun Protection Factor, but only for UVB. SPF is calculated by measuring how quickly your skin will burn with or without the sunscreen on. If you normally start to burn after twenty minutes, an SPF of 10 will supposedly keep you from burning for 200 minutes. SPF is also based on using a lot of sunscreen—like at least a teaspoon just for your face! Figure about an ounce for the rest of your body. That's a *lot*, too.

Sunscreen with physical blockers works right away. Sunscreen with chemical blockers needs at least twenty minutes to activate. I use sunscreen every day, rain or shine, and put it on right after I brush my teeth in the morning so I won't forget. I look absolutely ridiculous at the beach or pool because I am wearing a rash guard, shorts, a *huge* visor, *and* sunglasses. Even if people think I look like I'm wearing a turtleneck in the pool, who cares! Laugh on—I will be thankful in twenty years!

If you have kids, the best sunscreen for them is the kind you can actually get on them! If they don't like the smell, feel, packaging, or color—forget it! The point is to protect them as best we can and get them in the habit of protecting their skin themselves. There are a lot of fun options, from sticks to sprays to colorful, sparkly mermaid gels, and sun-protective clothing is a game changer, too! Rash guards are adorable, unisex, and carry a high SPF. My favorites are from J.Crew.

Also, sunscreen isn't exactly the most stable product. Heat is its enemy. If you keep it stashed in places that get very hot—inside your car, in your beach bag, in the bathroom—it will start to degrade and be less effective.

When You'll See Results

If you don't get any color or spots when you're outside, sunscreen worked that day, at least for UVB protection. But you can't know how well it protected you from UVA, as that damage takes place over decades.

Ingredients to Look For

For UVA chemical blockers: avobenzone, benzophenone, Mexoryl SX and XL.

For UVB chemical blockers: homosalate, octisalate, Tinosorb M and S.

For physical blockers: titanium dioxide, zinc oxide.

AVOID: octinoxate (allergic reactions), oxybenzone (hormone disruption), parabens (toxic), retinyl palmitate (DNA damage).

Stop Using This If

You get burned after very short sun exposure or your skin gets irritated or breaks out. Try a different brand.

Self-Tanners

Meant to Do

Grab one of these for a sun-kissed glow without risking any skin damage.

How It Works

The active ingredient in a self-tanner is a compound called DHA, or dihydroxyacetone, derived from sugar. It stains the dead skin cells on the top layer of your skin.

When You'll See Results

You should see some color right away. Many products take a few hours to deepen in tone. You'll always get the best results if you exfoliate with a gentle scrub before, because this will remove the topmost layer of dead skin cells, and the self-tanner will adhere better to the less-dead cells underneath.

Ingredients to Look For

DHA or tyrosine.

Stop Using This If

Your skin gets irritated or if you see any changes in the color of your urine. DHA is FDA-approved and safe for external use only. If your pee changes color, you might have applied too much DHA and it's getting into your system and being excreted by your kidneys. This rarely happens, but if it does, it warrants a speedy trip to the doctor!

◇◇◇◇◇◇◇◇◇◇◇◇◇◇◇◇◇◇◇◇

Next up, the doctor is in! Terry answers all the questions you've always wanted to ask, and some you didn't even *know* to ask! What to do, when to do it, does it work? Read on . . .

CHAPTER
5

You <u>Don't</u> Need the Knife : Nonsurgical MD Treatments and Procedures Guide

When I started my practice as a plastic surgeon, a patient's options were limited. A face with skin that was sagging? Get a facelift. Skin that needed rejuvenation? Get a deep chemical peel, which meant pain that left you howling; oozing, lipstick-red skin that looked so awful you didn't want to leave the house for weeks; and fears that your healing might leave you uneven or scarred. Do I miss those days? No way!

Thanks to the terrific trio of Botox, fillers, and lasers, it's now so much easier, less painful, and more affordable to find the right treatment—one that should leave you looking like yourself, only better. More refreshed and rejuvenated. Not like a shiny plastic bauble with cheeks so puffed out you'd think a bag of marshmallows was lodged in them. Or lips so engorged you'd think they'd split if the unfortunate victim tried to blow you a kiss.

Avoid at all costs what I call the "doesn't exist in nature" look—that weird, unnatural appearance due to improperly done procedures. Patients look almost as if they'd arrived in a spaceship and are searching for where they parked it.

What causes this? It all has to do with facial proportions. Typically, the facial width between the mid-pupils is half of the entire width of the mid-face. Got that? So if the mid-facial width becomes too wide due to overzealous filler injections, then you start to look like a sea creature rather than a rejuvenated and esthetically pleasing human being.

In addition to botched proportions, there are new-generation lasers and radio-frequency devices designed to nonsurgically tighten skin, but if they are used incorrectly, they can leave you scarred or with pigmentation changes (too dark or unevenly lightened spots) afterward. You need a deft hand to wield these devices!

I'll discuss this more in the next chapter, but you need to be very particular about who does your work. You should only go to board-certified dermatologists or plastic surgeons who have extensive experience doing the kind of treatment for which you're paying. The last thing you want is to get botched because a newbie or poorly trained technician hit the wrong setting on a laser.

Remember, a plastic surgeon can do injections of things like Botox and fillers, but a dermatologist *can't* do major surgical procedures like facelifts or implants. They might be excellent practitioners, but they also might want to talk you into procedures they *can* do (like fillers) when surgery might be a better option.

The treatments in this chapter are terrific options if you want to tackle anti-aging concerns like fine lines and wrinkles, loss of elasticity, hyperpigmentation, scarring, and, of course, Heather's hated cellulite. Always make sure to get the go-ahead from your physician if you have any underlying medical issues. The better your health, the better your results. Stop smoking. Exercise regularly. And have realistic expectations!

Botox

Stick a poison in your face to freeze your muscles? Fantastic, right? Botox was originally FDA-approved to treat eye muscle disorders, and when the FDA finally approved it for glabellar lines (those annoying frown lines between the eyebrows that make people look mad, sad, or old before their time) in 2002, shouts of hallelujah were heard from aging starlets as well as doctors who realized they were sitting on a non-insurance-reimbursable cash cow. Now, it's used to smooth foreheads and other wrinkles, and when done properly, it's amazingly rejuvenating.

What It Does

Botox is a trade name for Allergan Inc.'s botulinum toxin, a highly purified protein produced by the *Clostridium botulinum* bacterium. It works by blocking the nerve impulses that signal muscles to move. No movement of the muscles under the skin means no wrinkling of the skin above them.

The purified Botox is so unbelievably potent that the botulinum toxin dosage is measured in what's called "mouse units." In other words, one unit is equal to the amount that will kill 50 percent of a group of Swiss Webster mice when injected. Isn't that charming? A lethal dose of Botox for humans is approximately three thousand units. A standard Botox injection for glabellar, or frown lines, ranges from twenty-five up to about one hundred units, so it's not remotely toxic.

How It's Done

Botox comes in a fine powder that the doctor reconstitutes with sterile water. Once mixed, a very fine needle called a 30 gauge is used to inject the Botox.

Realistic Expectations

Botox can be a marvel when used properly; ridiculous when overdone. Doubtless you've seen a freakishly frozen and lineless forehead completely at odds with the rest of that person's face, which is not the look *you* ever want. It's not only guaranteed to make you look unnaturally smooth and strange, but *older* when you're trying to look younger. Too much Botox can also cause your eyebrows to raise way up in the dreaded look of surprise, or it can create a strangely shiny and bulging forehead.

It's important to do what we plastic surgeons call judicious Botox injections: appropriate, leaning toward conservative, to avoid the oddly frozen look that in people with high hairlines makes them look particularly cue-ballish. The general rule is that Botox injections are done from the nose up, and filler injections from the lips down.

Your expectations should be pretty minimal—that your wrinkles will be smoothed out. You should see results within a few days. Generally, Botox can only work well on moderately deep wrinkles. If they are too deep or too superficial, then the addition of a filler may be needed on certain parts of the face. Basically if your lines get worse with what we call "animation," meaning they are worse with facial expression or movement, then Botox will help.

Pain Meter

You might feel a little prick, but Botox injections should not be painful and don't need numbing with a topical anesthetic beforehand. Ice placed on the skin or an expertly done "distraction" maneuver makes Botox injections nearly painless.

Recuperation Time

None, really. You just need to keep your head upright for a few hours after the injections so the Botox molecule doesn't spread to unintended areas like the upper eyelid muscles.

Possible Complications/What Can Go Wrong

Sometimes new patients complain to me that they had Botox with someone else and they didn't see any changes at all. I explain that once the Botox is mixed and placed in the injectable solution, the efficacy clock starts clicking. For every day it sits in solution un-injected, it starts to lose its potency. The fresher, the better. Within about two weeks, it becomes weakly effective. Old, over-diluted Botox is probably the number one reason your Botox didn't work.

I have been fortunate to have accumulated many years of experience doing Botox injections. Injecting Botox is an art. It's not paint by numbers. You have to take the arch of the brows, the shape of the forehead, a patient's age, and especially how lax their skin is into consideration. Inject too much or in the wrong places and the forehead can droop. Inject it too close to the eyebrow and it drops your brows and gives you a heavy "lidded" look. Inject too close to the eyes and that can result in a very disturbing droopy eyelid that can last for several weeks. This is called ptosis and it's not that rare when Botox is done by an inexperienced injector. If that happens, you need special eyedrops called Iopidine, used every four hours, to correct the problem.

I also see people with these weirdly shiny foreheads—it's something to do with the sweat glands being paralyzed, which is why Botox can be used in the armpits for those who have an excessive sweat problem. A shiny forehead is a telltale giveaway that they're doing too much.

Occasionally we will inject Botox in the lip area for deep-expression smile lines but unless it's perfectly done, it may leave you looking, at worst, like a stroke victim. Not the exact look we are going for here!

Another common complication is that Botox can make your eyelid twitch. This has nothing to do with the skill of the doctor—it just happens. I know, because when Heather and I were about to get married in 1999, we were driving to Palm Springs and it happened to her!

Picture this: The top's down and the wind is in our hair. I'm so happy and so in love and so excited. It was a wonderful day. I'd injected Heather two weeks earlier for the wedding photos, and I suddenly noticed that she was starting to get a droopy eyelid. I was at the wheel so I couldn't stare at her to figure it out. Maybe, I told myself, I was just imagining things. I didn't want her to get worried or paranoid. And then I saw her eye twitch some more and all I could think was, this is going to get worse and still be like that for our wedding and it was all my fault.

"'Why do you keep looking at me?," Heather said after a few minutes. "Is something wrong with my eye? It feels funny."

"Don't worry," I told her. "You just need some eyedrops."

Luckily, Iopidine, the eyedrops I already mentioned, also works on twitching. Fortunately, the drops worked on Heather and our wedding and all the photos went off without a hitch, but trust me—it's the last thing you want to happen!

This brings me to two more points that aren't medical complications but *esthetic* complications. This first is, how "frozen" do you want to look? You must discuss this with your doctor. If you're looking for a very deep frozen look, it will take a lot more Botox, and the complication rate goes up along with the price of the injections. The second is that people often end up looking so frozen because they figured it's better to save a little money and go to someone unqualified than to pay for the best they can afford at the practice of a highly experienced cosmetic dermatologist or plastic surgeon. Buyer beware.

You should also know that Botox has a fixed price to physicians. As you read above, it comes in a powder form, and we dilute it. If someone is offering Botox at bargain basement prices, it's probably being made in a basement, and you'll have zero control over its strength and purity. Is that what you want to have injected into your skin? Worse, doctors who may be great gynecologists or internists (but not experienced with injectables), as well as quacks who are "Botox party" purveyors, may think they know what they're doing, but they rarely have had the training cosmetic dermatologists and surgeons possess. You don't want to be on the wrong end of their needles!

Lasts For

This is the big catch with Botox. It's temporary. This is good if you went to a quack; bad if you're looking refreshed and rejuvenated and you watch those effects wear off. Expect it to last for three to six months, although if you get regular injections it does last a bit longer. Also, with prolonged use, you may develop antibodies that reduce Botox's effectiveness. If so, you need to switch to one of the other neurotransmitter molecules like Xeomin or Dysport that have a slightly different structure and will not have the same reaction.

Cellulite Treatments

As you know already, cellulite is hereditary, stubborn, and really tough to treat. The problem is that there's no one treatment that is uniformly effective. You can try wraps, Endermologie, radiotherapy, liposuction, or lasers,

Heather: I'm obsessed with getting rid of cellulite. It's a genetic th
something I've had to deal with since puberty. I have tried every
and every treatment ever put on the market. When I was a teenage
to take the train into Manhattan to a salon for body wraps. It was th
the Hollywood stars went to for perfect, camera-ready bodies. You'
there naked in total mortification, and they'd take gauze that was dre
in some special, secret solution and wrap you like a mummy. Did it
Temporarily. As in, for a day or two.

Years later, did I learn my lesson? No, I did not. I once stupidly wen
course of mesotherapy, which was the hottest thing in France but is ille
this country. And it should be. It's injections in your butt and legs tha
allegedly vitamins but are actually medically unapproved and really po
ful chemicals that cause inflammation. I went four times and got so s
had to take antinausea meds. Was it worth it? Of course not—and I'm lu
didn't have serious complications or infections. It's much safer to stick v
a treatment like the wraps I did in New York City as a teenager or Enderm
gie, which we'll describe below.

but no treatment is guaranteed to give you either partial or permane
results.

What It Does

Endermologie causes temporary swelling, which minimizes the
appearance of cellulite without actually breaking it up and getting rid
of it. It causes local cells to leak fluid, and this fluid can cause thickening and swelling of the skin, temporarily reducing the appearance of
cellulite.

How It's Done

Rollers are applied to the cellulite, usually for an hour. A series of
weekly or biweekly treatments are done to prolong the effects. After a
few weeks you can start to see subtle improvements, but they will fade
quickly once you stop the treatments.

Realistic Expectations

As cellulite is so stubborn, having low expectations is always wise.

Pain Meter

Mild discomfort, like a deep tissue massage.

Recuperation Time

None.

Possible Complications/What Can Go Wrong

A lot of bruising and soreness, but overall very well tolerated.

Lasts For

A few weeks if you're very lucky. After your initial sessions, you need to have at least monthly treatments in perpetuity to keep seeing results.

Dermabrasion and Microdermabrasion

What It Does

Dermabrasion is strictly old school. It's a tricky procedure where a diamond burr is used to scrape off the top layers of skin. It's effective, but the tricky part comes during the healing afterward. Those with fair skin could expect to be red and blotchy for weeks if not months; those with dark skin never could predict if their skin would fully recover an even tone—if it was mottled, it was permanent.

Except for treating extremely deep scars, I don't recommend dermabrasion anymore, because lasers give me so much more control over how many layers of skin to remove. Microdermabrasion is a much better way to go when you want to improve your skin's texture and promote collagen production. The only problem is that results are very limited at best.

How It's Done

Again, dermabrasion scrapes off the top layers of skin with a diamond burr. Microdermabrasion gently exfoliates by applying fine jet crystals directly to the face, which removes dead skin cells.

Realistic Expectations

Dermabrasion: dramatic wrinkle reduction but great risk of skin pigment loss or gain, with a great potential for hypo- (lighter) or hyperpigmentation (darker). Microdermabrasion: minimal skin texture improvements with essentially no risk.

Pain Meter

Dermabrasion needs general anesthesia. Microdermabrasion causes zero pain.

Recuperation Time

With dermabrasion, you'll spend seven to ten days looking like a monster. Microdermabrasion needs no recuperation. You can have a treatment and go right back to work.

Possible Complications/What Can Go Wrong

With dermabrasion, there is a high risk for scarring and pigmentation issues—dark or light spots and blotches, which are permanent. There are no complications with microdermabrasion unless your practitioner is a complete quack.

Lasts For

Dermabrasion lasts for years; microdermabrasion lasts for weeks.

Fat Transfer

Just as I never imagined that someday I'd be injecting a purified poison into my patients' foreheads to smooth out their wrinkles, I never thought that injecting fat into their faces or butts would be so popular, either.

What It Does

Fat transfer is done with your own body fat so there's no risk of a reaction to it. By injecting it into certain areas, volume is increased. In your face, it's realistically increased. In your butt, the sky seems to be the limit. This is referred to as the Brazilian butt lift—and it's out of control. Literally and unfortunately!

How It's Done

Fat is removed from one or two areas of your body (usually the stomach and outer thighs), processed, and put into precise injection syringes for transfer. In the face, it's best to overcorrect (inject more fat) by 10 to 20 percent to account for natural absorption; in the buttocks, as much as 40 percent or more can reabsorb.

Realistic Expectations

In the 1970s it was all about the small butt. Then in the 1980s it became, "Does this dress make my butt look big?" Now, it's "I really hope these pants make my butt look big." Blame it on a change in our esthetics, but expecting to go from a normal-sized butt to an enormous one with your own fat is a crapshoot.

Pain Meter

I had a patient whose facial fat transfer was done by a celebrity dermatologist. She had a dose of Valium and was relaxed and happy until the doctor accidentally hit, literally, a nerve, and this patient practically jumped off the table. A short while later, when the fat was ready to be injected, a topical anesthetic cream was applied to her face, but this patient was still in shock from the unexpected jolt of pain, and getting the needles in her face was agony.

Be warned. Fat is a thick substance, so the syringes used to inject it can't be as fine as those used for Botox or some of the other fillers. The butt is far less sensitive than the face, so it's not as painful. Most of my patients only need a little Valium on board to tolerate the treatment, and a little local anesthetic done pre-injection.

Recuperation Time

For the face, you might be a little sore and bruised at the injection sites, but icing and an OTC painkiller are all you need. For butts, since a very large amount of fat is injected (up to one liter per cheek), a much longer, painful recovery is characterized by you needing to sit on a foam donut for ten days and take significant doses of high-strength pain pills for three to five days.

Possible Complications/What Can Go Wrong

Season three of *Botched* was all about the butt; nothing but butt complications. That's because doing a moderate butt augmentation (a range of 300–500 cc of fat) is a pretty reliable, low-risk procedure. But I can' t tell you how many cases I've seen where the augmentation was way, way higher than that. What happens afterward? How about a whopping dose of a flesh-eating disease, called necrotizing fasciitis, caused by bacteria? If you do get this condition, you will need to have all the muscles cut out of the area and undergo soft tissue and skin grafts. This is incredibly painful and disfiguring and potentially lethal. And for what? For a bigger butt that no reputable surgeon would advise you to have.

One *Botched* patient I had went to a plastic surgeon well known for buttock augmentation—but it turned out that he was a gynecologist. Her consultation was scheduled for a Thursday at two in the afternoon, and he said, "You're in luck; I have an opening today." So, two hours later he did the fat transfer and it was a disaster. He put way too much in and her butt looked bizarre and misshapen. She says he told her to *gain* twenty pounds so he could put even more in and reshape it, and this time it was even worse. When she came to see me I had to suction it, which is something you normally don't do on a buttock because it can lose its shape; it's not like breasts, which are more easily malleable. And you can't put scars everywhere because there are no areas on the buttock to effectively hide the incisions.

This patient learned the hard way that doctors often won't tell you up front that if you want a really big butt, you might need to gain twenty or thirty pounds . . . but even with that volume of fat, you're not going to be guaranteed that it'll last. And because you're reinjecting your own fat, you're not going to be losing any pounds during the procedure. You can be risking your health with that kind of weight gain just to have a big booty.

Lasts For

It's impossible to know how much of the fat will stick. Sometimes, as much as 40 percent or more will be absorbed back into your body and there is absolutely no way to stop this from happening.

Fillers

Hit the beach too many times? Smoked a few too many cigarettes? Drove a convertible to work for years on congested and polluted highways? Lived through a ton of stress? Or just gotten older? All of the above cause wrinkles, sagging, and a loss of fullness in our faces and make you a candidate for injectable fillers. They're extremely popular because they are noninvasive, quick, and well tested, and they work. They can pretty much enhance almost any area of your face, and make you feel a lot more confident about your appearance.

What It Does

Fillers add volume to the skin to diminish the appearance of wrinkles and creases, and eliminate hollows and a sunken-in look on your face.

How It's Done

The filler is injected under your skin with a syringe. Depending on how deep the wrinkles and how large the area, you could need one or more syringes, and different kinds of fillers for different kinds of lines. These are the most commonly used fillers that I recommend (except the last one):

❖ Juvederm is made from hyaluronic acid, a naturally occurring substance found in every cell, and is used to add volume, especially around the nose and mouth, in the lips, and in the hollows under the eyes. It's also good for severe facial wrinkles and creases.

❖ Perlane is made from a hyaluronic acid similar to Restylane, and is best for smile lines and to plump up lips.

❖ Prevelle Silk is made from hyaluronic acid and is used to restore fullness to the face and lips.

❖ Radiesse is a safe alternative to collagen (which I don't use anymore, as it caused too many allergic reactions and was very short-lasting). It not only fills in wrinkles and provides volume to the face, but it also stimulates the body to produce collagen. It is most often used to treat the cheeks, the area below the eyes, the nasolabial folds (the lines around the nose and mouth), the marionette lines (from the corners of your mouth down to your jawline), the creases at the corners of your mouth, pre-jowl lines, chin wrinkles, acne scars, and deep depressions in the face.

❖ Zestylane is made from hyaluronic acid and is used most often for moderate to severe wrinkles in the cheeks, other facial areas like the marionette lines, the nasolabial folds, and in and around the lips. All hyaluronic acid injections have the added benefit of being reversible with the use of hyaluronidase, an enzyme that breaks down hyaluronic acid in seconds. It can be used at any point after a hyaluronic acid injection, so time is not an issue.

❖ Sculptra is made from poly-L-lactic acid and is used in the hollow areas of the temples and the mid-cheek area. It is not to be used in the thin skin of the eyes, as it can cause permanent nodules to form, or directly in the nasolabial folds. It improves fullness by inducing long-lasting (up to three years) collagen stimulation. I think its super effective for when the temple and mid-face areas are losing facial volume as you age and you start to look skeletonized, or what we call cadaveric.

❖ Silicone is a permanent filler normally used in breast implants, and I do not recommend it. It's too tricky to control, you can react badly to it, and surgery is the only way to remove it. It's also illegal unless done in a micro-droplet form, which is very risky. Basically, don't do it, please. I'm busy enough as it is fishing out scarred tissue destroyed by free silicone injections.

Realistic Expectations

When new plastic surgery procedures are developed so you can have a *new* new face, there is a general rule you should know: we tend to overdo things until we figure them out. Never has this been truer than with injectable fillers.

What do you think when some actresses appear with cheeks so puffed out they make chipmunks look like they'd just had liposuction? Or when so many people seem to have these bizarrely homogenized facial proportions that don't look as if they exist in nature—because they *don't*? They don't just look bizarre—worse, they look *fake*.

That's why I keep saying that the enemy of good is *better*. A lot of people want the whole enchilada: they want the most for their money, they don't want to come in for regular appointments, and they want things to last—which I totally understand, of course—so they ask to be over-filled. Their dermatologists or plastic surgeons don't want to lose the patient and they agree to do what the patient is requesting for fear of losing them to the doctor down the hall or across the street. Penny-wise, pound-foolish!

Also, if you get over-filled and get used to it, it's like rewiring your brain to accept something as pleasing or as "normal" when you might have thought differently about it at first. As Heather says, how many of us grew up thinking that enormously puffy lips were aspirational? Who *really* wants duck lips?

So, your expectations should be that you'll look less wrinkled and/or droopy, yet still like *you*. You do not want to be so over-filled that you look as plump as a turkey butt, or gotten botched so your face is lumpy and uneven. My advice is to limit yourself to one or at the very most two syringes of filler. Let it settle in and then reassess. And always, *always* go to a skilled injector with lots of experience.

Pain Meter

Some of my patients are so happy to get filler that they don't mind the needle sticks. Others are so phobic and tense that they need some Valium before the appointment. The pain factor is mild, but certain areas around the nose and lips can be really sensitive.

Recuperation Time

There is limited downtime after your treatment, but do not do it within a few days of an important event in your life because you probably will be a bit red, swollen, and/or bruised around some of the injection sites for a few days to a few weeks. Icing right after the injections can help. Anything more serious is rare and warrants an immediate call to your practitioner.

Possible Complications/What Can Go Wrong

Recently, two dreaded complications have come to light regarding excessive filler injecting, and you need to know about them because fillers are often sold as harmless, with zero complications, and that's just not true.

The first complication is necrosis. Necrosis is skin death. Once it's dead, it can't be revived. Filler is commonly injected around the naso-labial folds, and when done properly, you'll look great. But we're not supposed to inject Radiesse in the central third of the face, around your nose and eyes, because of the chance it will block the main artery bringing blood to your nose. If that happens, you can lose all the skin on your nose or cheek. The protocol to try to reverse this (usually with anti-inflammatory steroids) doesn't work all that well, either. Or, if filler is injected incorrectly, it can block the blood supply to the entire territory of your face. If that happens, and the blood supply can't adequately oxygenate the area, you can get skin necrosis of your entire face.

The second serious potential complication is blindness. It's rare, but not *so* rare—which means it's listed on our consent forms, just as death is listed on consent forms whenever you're having surgery. We don't list it because we *expect* it to occur, but because there is still a remote possibility.

Why? There are facial blood vessels that track back into the optic region near your retina, and these provide the blood supply to that part of the face. If a non-dissolvable filler inadvertently gets into blood vessels that supply the optic nerve with blood and oxygen, especially around the retina, due to the way the arteries in this area are formed,

What If You're Needle-Phobic?

If you are a low-pain threshold, sensitive, and needle-phobic person (who isn't, really?), then good preparation is the key. Have your doctor give you a pre-visit dose of Valium, which will relax you. Use lots of ice, and tell your doctor to distract you with gentle taps from the other hand. Better yet, go to an experienced doctor with a good bedside manner who will be sensitive to your understandable needle phobia. Anyone who downplays it or tells you "It doesn't hurt" when it really does is not a very good doctor!

it has nowhere to go—and the blindness clock starts ticking. What's really scary is that you can go blind from injections done rather far away from the eye; in the forehead or lower cheek areas, for example.

So if you have filler in your face and suddenly notice blurry vision or worse, it is an absolute *medical emergency* and you need treatment within an hour or two or you could become permanently blinded in that eye. Restylane can be dissolved, but permanent fillers like silicone need a surgeon to try to minimize the damage. This is yet another reason why you need an experienced physician to do your injections to ensure that none of the filler is going to end up in a blood vessel.

If you're worried after reading this, you should be. Complications can happen to even the very best and most experienced doctors, but your chances of them are so much smaller if you choose your practitioner wisely. You need to be a smart shopper when you're planning to have foreign substances injected into your face!

Lasts For

The fillers I recommend are all temporary, and their longevity depends on the type you choose as well as your unique facial characteristics and skin quality. That said, most fillers will gradually disappear within six months to a year. In particular:

- ❖ Juvederm: six to eight months
- ❖ Perlane: eight to ten months
- ❖ Prevelle Silk: three months
- ❖ Radiesse: about one year
- ❖ Restylane: six to nine months
- ❖ Sculptra: one to three years

And I already know you would never, ever consider getting a permanent filler in your face!

Lasers

Lasers are amazing devices that give you an effective and non-invasive way to rejuvenate, resurface, and/or tighten your skin. I love that, in many cases, they've also replaced the need for many of the older procedures, such as heavy-duty chemical peels or dermabrasion, to make you look a lot younger with far less risk.

Lasers can diminish facial lines and wrinkles, blemishes, skin discolorations, and even minor scarring. They used to only be able to effectively treat fair or medium skin tones, since they sometimes left darker patches or unevenness on darker skin tones, but they've become increasingly sophisticated and better suited to everyone. It's all very Star Trek, and as the technology improves, the accuracy and effectiveness go up and the risks go down. Discuss your options with your dermatologist or plastic surgeon. You absolutely can't compare your skin to anyone else's, as your skin tone and texture will always be unique to you.

What It Does

Lasers generate invisible infrared light, whose wavelength is matched to the cell it's designed to target. For skin resurfacing, it targets the epithelial (skin) cells, delivering specific targeted energy designed to ablate or destroy the skin cell. For discoloration or pigmentation problems, the laser will have a wavelength matching the clot of the pigment cell exactly, directing energy only to that cell and sparing the other cells located in the skin.

How It's Done

The handset of the laser is passed over your skin, targeting the specific area you want treated.

Fraxel is one of the most commonly used and effective lasers to reverse the signs of aging by stimulating the production of collagen. It also improves the appearance of imperfections, including fine lines and wrinkles, such as crow's feet and brow lines; acne scars and other surface scars; discolorations and age spots; sun damage; and precancerous lesions, such as actinic keratosis (which commonly appear on the forehead as pinkish or dark splotches). Each treatment takes about fifteen to forty-five minutes. Usually the procedure is done after applying numbing cream for at least forty-five minutes, and a light sedative is sometimes used, too.

The Fx CO_2 laser treats the deeper layers by stimulating collagen production and replacing damaged skin with new, fresh skin. This improves the appearance of fine lines and wrinkles, deep frown lines, and skin tone and texture. Each treatment typically takes less than an hour to complete. Most cases require very deep sedation or general anesthesia.

For hair removal, first your skin will get numbed with a topical anesthetic. Then the handheld laser device is pressed directly on your skin to deliver pulses of light energy. This energy is powerful enough to destroy the deepest part of the hair follicle but gentle enough to not disturb the surrounding tissues. Treatment may take several minutes to several hours to complete, depending on the size and number of areas. The newer state-of-the-art laser hair removal devices use a suction device to minimize the distance between the laser beam and the skin, reducing the pain level to almost zero.

Realistic Expectations

For skin rejuvenation, lasers are one of my favorite go-to treatments. Although there will be a noticeable improvement after just one treatment, you almost always need multiple treatments over a period of a year for the best results, depending on the severity of the condition treated.

In other words, lasers are fantastic rejuvenators, but they're not total miracle workers if you want to treat conditions like deep wrinkling, tattoos, pigmentation problems, and certain diseases like rosacea (skin reddening) or rhinophyma (coarsening of the skin on the nose).

For hair removal, lasers can only work on dark hair, ideally on light or medium complexions. Because you have so many hair follicles in different stages of resting/growth, you'll likely need several treatments for optimal results, usually over a span of three months. It's important to understand that laser hair removal is called permanent hair *reduction*. Periodic touch-ups will be required yearly or every other year.

Pain Meter

Skin rejuvenation lasers always need some form of numbing, either with topical anesthesia or, in some cases, with general anesthesia (which always has a risk factor but means you won't feel a thing).

Laser hair removal usually isn't painful unless you're working in extremely sensitive parts of the body like the upper lip or pubic area, where it can hurt a lot. Because the process is so quick, pain is usually extremely well tolerated.

Recuperation Time

Laser procedures that are minimally invasive require little to no downtime, and you can have the procedure done at lunchtime and go right back to work afterward and resume your normal activities. For rejuvenation with the Fx CO_2 laser, however, you will probably see some mild crusting, swelling, and bruising that will last for as long as a week, but usually you can be seen in public between three to five days after treatment. This happens with the Fx CO_2 laser since it goes deeper, but as it treats only a fraction of your skin at a time, leaving a lot of untouched skin in between the lasered areas, it speeds up healing.

You *must* stay out of the sun after any laser treatment, since new layers of skin have been exposed and you can easily get burned—which could lead to a much longer recuperation time, treatment for the burn, and the kind of skin damage you were trying to undo in the first place!

Possible Complications/What Can Go Wrong

Lasers are not toys. They can do serious damage. In inexperienced hands they can cause serious scarring, pigmentation problems, and blotchy skin issues that are nearly impossible to fix. In fact, as a certified medical-legal expert for the Medical Board of California, I can tell you that laser hair removal, which is a speedy and relatively straightforward procedure, is still the single most common cause of a malpractice lawsuit among all laser and all cosmetic treatments, including major plastic surgery procedures.

There are a lot of storefront laser centers all over America now, and you need to make sure that whoever's holding that laser wand has had extensive experience before they aim it at your vulnerable skin. Lasers are what we call Class 5 devices, which means they are potentially dangerous enough that only doctors or a trained nurse directly under the supervision of the doctor can use them. However, it's been reported that untrained individuals who aren't doctors or supervised nurses are doing laser treatments in all fifty states. Buyer beware! This is at best illegal and at worst incredibly dangerous.

Even with the proper credentials, laser operators may not know who exactly are the appropriate candidates for laser treatments. This is especially worrisome for those with darker skin tones, as these individuals have very active melanocytes, the cells responsible for making pigment, and lasers applied inappropriately can cause severe hyperpigmentation, with dark blotches or streaks over the entire face. If that doesn't convince you to have a trained physician do your laser treatment, I don't know what will!

Lasts For

In most cases, the results of effective laser treatments will last for years if proper skin protection and maintenance are applied. Yes, that means sunscreen is numero uno on your list of musts-to-apply *every* day, unless there is a hurricane outside or you are not leaving the house!

Light Therapy

The category of light therapy—the most common is IPL, or intense pulsed light—is used for skin rejuvenation and to improve and/or even out skin tone. It works by applying energy in a similar manner to lasers, but these devices have wavelengths outside the range of lasers. This gives them the ability to deliver less potentially risky wavelengths to the skin, but because their energy is lower than that of lasers, it makes them less effective.

What It Does

Light therapy devices target the cells called chromophores, which contain certain pigments that give them color.

How It's Done

Similar to a laser, a hand piece connects to the light box's energy source and is passed over your skin.

Realistic Expectations

You can expect to see less redness, better skin tone, and a reduction in pigmentation problems.

Pain Meter

It can be negligible for the gentlest treatments, and then range up to moderate, depending on severity of the problem.

Recuperation Time

Almost none.

Possible Complications/What Can Go Wrong

See lasers, as the possible complications are the same—mainly scarring, hyperpigmentation, and hypopigmentation.

Lasts For

It can last for months to a year, depending on your skincare and exposure to the sun. Hint: Always use sunscreen, and with a high SPF, especially in the weeks after your treatment.

Liposuction

As we get older, it takes more and more hard work to keep our weight steady and our muscles strong. Gravity is a bitch, all right—but it has nothing to do with the physiological fact that as your hormone levels naturally decline with age, your body's propensity to hold onto fat increases. It's not fair, but you can do something about it—at least *some* people can do something in *some* areas of the body. This is what liposuction is for.

What It Does

Anyone who works out diligently should know that you can do a gazillion crunches every day, but exercise *can't* actually spot-reduce fat in your belly or any particular area of your body. (Don't believe anyone who says it does—it can make your muscles larger and stronger, but it can't reduce *fat*.) Liposuction is the *only* procedure that can specifically remove fat cells from targeted areas of your body. It removes fat from love handles and muffin tops in the abdomen; "bat wings" or jiggly upper arms; the area around the frame of the buttocks (but almost never the butt cheek itself); the inner thighs and the saddlebags of the outer thighs; and calves and ankles.

How It's Done

A small incision is made in the skin, numbing medicine called tumescent fluid is injected, and the fat is aspirated or suctioned out.

Realistic Expectations

Liposuction is *not* a weight-loss procedure and it is *not* helpful if your skin is very loose. It works best for people who have stubborn fat deposits in specific areas who are close to their ideal body weight, who exercise regularly and have good muscle tone, and who eat a healthy

A Few Words About Pain

Everyone has a different pain threshold and sensitivities, but I've found that most of the procedures I do cause minimal pain. Many patients are willing to endure it because they know the benefits outweigh the discomfort. (On the other hand, I've done thousands of liposuctions with local anesthesia, and every once in a while I can't get the patient numb or they're so sensitive and so anxious that any little touch causes a reaction.)

The biggest issue is underestimating how much pain there can be post-procedure, especially after surgery. For many years, we in American medicine have claimed that these procedures require very little recovery and produce very little pain, which isn't necessarily true. What I tell patients is it's like a bell curve, with standard deviations. Some people will feel basically nothing and some people will experience horrible pain—and then there's everybody else in between. The shock of severe pain can actually intensify how bad you're hurting, which is why I am blunt and exaggerate the pain potential with everyone, just so they know!

Don't try and macho it out when you're in pain. Follow your doctor's orders. I prescribe painkillers very liberally the first couple of weeks after surgery so patients can control their pain and heal. Pain control is a really important part of the recovery process.

---

diet. In other words, they've done everything right, but their bodies are built to hold on to fat in certain places, such as the outer thighs or buttocks. Let me repeat this: liposuction is *not* a weight-loss procedure!

What happens, though, is that liposuction is offered to pretty much everyone who asks for it, even if they are not ideal candidates or want to lose weight (even if they say they don't!). Liposuction can work extremely well or it can work sort of well. No matter what your weight—and you can be of medium weight or even a bit heavy, as long as you're strong and healthy—it's all about your skin's elasticity and how well you heal. You absolutely must have realistic expectations, as no one can predict how well your body will respond to liposuction.

Sometimes, too, what you really need is a more invasive treatment, such as a tummy tuck if your abdominal skin is loose enough and your muscles have separated due to pregnancy. But if the practitioner you're consulting doesn't do tucks, and if you've already said you want liposuction, believe me, you're going to be offered the liposuction. That will be a waste of time, money, and pain. Not only that, but it can make your skin looser and look far worse after surgery than before.

Also, liposuction is *never* recommended for cellulite—removing some of the fat can actually make it worse and lumpier.

Pain Meter

During the procedure, you will have local anesthesia and IV sedation or general anesthesia, so you won't feel a thing. Afterward, you will be very bruised, swollen, and in pain, although some areas of the body (like the abdominal area) hurt worse than others. You will need to wear compression garments for several weeks.

Recuperation Time

You should start to feel less achy after a few days, but expect discomfort for four to six weeks. After that, recuperation is swift, but you will not be able to exercise or do any lifting for at least six weeks after the procedure.

Possible Complications/What Can Go Wrong

I've seen patients who had liposuction on their thighs and then gained a lot of weight. Sure, the fat cells had been removed from their legs—but the fat from their weight gain had to go somewhere. So it showed up in unsightly places like their bellies and upper arms.

As with lasers, a lot of practitioners take a weekend training course and then start offering liposuction. This is not a good idea. It's a full-blown surgical procedure, and while it's not difficult, you still want to know you are in capable hands. I've seen a lot of patients on *Botched* whose liposuction went terribly wrong. The complications can be mild, such as skin loosening, but can also be severe, leaving patients with extreme contour irregularities, punctured organs beneath the skin, and even death.

I need you to think of liposuction as something as potentially serious as a heart attack. It should *never* be approached casually. It is one of the most common procedures in cosmetic surgery, and it also has one of the highest dissatisfaction rates. It goes badly all the time. It is absolutely imperative to not have significant skin laxity, and it must be done conservatively by a trained individual. The last thing you want is your family sobbing at your funeral because you wanted thinner thighs.

Lasts For

Liposuction should last for years, if not decades, as long as you maintain a stable weight. Pregnancy or weight gain can affect your results.

Peels

Chemical peels used to be truly terrifying. Before lasers became so effective, chemical peels were often the go-to treatment for skin rejuvenation, but the harsh acids used to peel off the skin sometimes did tremendous damage.

What It Does

Peels are a noninvasive treatment where you deliberately damage the skin by removing the topmost layer so that fresh new skin replaces it. A mixture of different acids leaves skin smoother and firmer as they eliminate wrinkles, hyperpigmentation, and age spots.

How It's Done

There are three different levels of peels:

❖ Over-the-counter. OTC strength of AHAs (alpha hydroxy acids, including glycolic), up to 35 percent, which should be done by a trained esthetician.

❖ Medium peel. This uses trichloroacetic acid, Jessner's solution, or glycolic acid at a concentration of 50 to 70 percent.

❖ Deep peel. This uses phenol or Baker's solution. I don't recommend this, as phenol can cause heart damage, and medium peels and lasers are so much better! Never, ever do a medium or deep peel unless you are in the hands of a competent and experienced physician.

Realistic Expectations

Mild improvements only.

Pain Meter

Minimal for superficial peels. Deep peels sometimes require general anesthesia.

Recuperation Time

After the peel, your skin forms a sort of mask, which then peels off. Depending on how deep your peel, you can look pretty terrible (red and raw and oozing) during this process.

Possible Complications/What Can Go Wrong

Like lasers, scarring and pigmentation problems can occur.

Lasts For

Months to years.

Prescription Topicals

One of the best anti-aging treatments you can do is a very simple one. It's done with a prescription-only cream called Retin-A.

What It Does

Retin-A is a vitamin A derivative that strips excess dead skin cells off the top layer of your skin. It is also the only skincare ingredient that can stimulate collagen production—which means that it actually encourages your skin to renew itself. It can be used to repair sun damage, minimize age or hyperpigmentation spots, reduce wrinkles, and make your skin look healthier.

How It's Done

You apply the cream as directed by your doctor.

Realistic Expectations

With consistent use, Retin-A can greatly reduce fine lines and clear up pigmentation problems.

Pain Meter

There should never be any pain, but Retin-A can be intensely irritating when you first start using it, leaving your skin dry and flaky.

Recuperation Time

It's always best to start at a very low dose and gradually increase it as your skin learns to tolerate it. There are different formulations and strengths, so you might need to experiment until you find the best one. Most people have few problems with it.

Possible Complications/What Can Go Wrong

You absolutely must always wear a good, broad-spectrum sunscreen, as Retin-A makes your skin much more susceptible to burns. Not just little red splotches but serious, deep sunburns. Most people apply Retin-A at night, since you're even more susceptible to burns with a fresh dose on your face in the morning.

Lasts For

You can keep using Retin-A for years, but the effects will wear off if you stop regular use. There's no reason to stop, unless you have intolerable irritation. It really is a great rejuvenator.

Radiotherapy

With radiotherapy, radio waves supply energy to the superficial layers of the skin. The most common procedure is called Thermage.

What It Does

This treatment is used to tighten the skin, reducing the need for surgical skin-tucking procedures, such as a facelift or neck lift.

How It's Done

A radio frequency wand is passed over the skin, delivering the energy similar to how a laser wand is used.

Realistic Expectations

Radiotherapy is meant to stimulate collagen production in the deep layers of your skin, and induce tightening by using heat. My opinion is that it provides only mild skin tightening at best.

Pain Meter

This procedure is very painful, even with topical anesthesia, so I don't usually recommend it.

Recuperation Time

It can take several days for redness and swelling to go down.

Possible Complications/What Can Go Wrong

There can be scarring, burns, blisters, and prolonged nerve pain. It is also hard to predict how long the results will last.

Lasts For

Months at best.

◇◇◇◇◇◇◇◇◇◇◇◇◇◇◇◇◇◇

The key advice I can give anyone who wants to use modern technology to improve their appearance is to go into a consultation with a certain degree of skepticism. This is a business, after all, and whatever procedures or technology a doctor or wellness provider uses for revenue is going to pay for overhead, no matter how well it works or how skilled these practitioners are. If all a doctor has is a hammer, everything is going to look like a nail. Research carefully, speak to former patients, and spend the least amount of money you can to get the desired result. Be smart. Be educated. And be as frugal as possible.

6

You <u>Do</u> Need the Knife Plastic Surgery 101—How to Be a Smart Patient

Let me tell you something about cutting people open: It's *easy*. Yes, easy! It's not very complicated. And for me, it's *fun*.

Seriously! But here's the catch. Surgery is like tennis. Learning the sport is easy once you master the basics; *becoming* a great tennis player means hours of daily practice for *years*. Surgery is no different. Learning how to cut people open and sew them back up again is straightforward; doing it with a deft touch and becoming really good at it takes *years*. And, of course, the obvious difference is that if you botch your tennis game, no big deal. But if you botch someone's surgical procedure, the consequences can be dire. The patients could look awful. Or the patients could look even worse—because they're *dead*.

If you go to five different surgeons, what will you do if they recommend five completely different procedures? How do you know what's best? Which surgeon do you choose so you don't get botched? Read on for the inside scoop on how to find the right surgeon, what to expect, and what procedures are available so you can make the most informed choices possible.

Before we go on, however, I'm going to let you in on a very important secret. If you are *under the age of forty*, you do not need surgical anti-aging treatments.

If you could look inside the waiting rooms of every cosmetic derma-tologist and plastic surgeon in America, you might be astonished at how *young* the wannabe patients are. I mean, if you're not old enough to buy a drink, I don't think you're old enough to need breast augmentation, lipo-suction, or fillers.

Practically every week, I have kids who are sixteen and seventeen come in with their moms. They ask for fillers in their perfectly shaped cheeks and lips, and for implants in their perfectly fine and still-growing breasts. At that age! I tell them that teenagers or young adults who get a lot of work done often regret it a scant few years later. I explain that breast implants should only be considered after your breasts are fully developed, and usually not before the age of twenty-two, which is when the FDA has approved silicone implants. Then I send them away.

But the problem is that there will always be someone else who will agree to do what these patients want.

I think there are two reasons why plastic surgery patients are getting younger and younger. The first is peer pressure, especially thanks to social media. Heather and I discuss this all the time, because we know our kids (especially our three girls) and their friends are very vulnerable to this in a way we never were, because we mercifully grew up without the ability to instantly post photos of our every activity online. Her mom would have *plotzed* if Heather asked for lip filler, breast implants, or even Botox had they been available. We don't think any parent should allow body modifi-cation—and to us, lip or cheek filler falls into that category—in any of their children until the age of consent.

Plus, we know that models and celebrities—the role models young women often look up to—are given the Photoshop treatment, even though their skin might be flawless. It's still very hard for people of all ages to know what's real and what's fake. If you're already worried about your appearance or feeling down on yourself, seeing all these idealized images can make you even more insecure. In reality, of course, these images are ridiculously unobtainable.

The second reason is that greed has warped a lot of this industry. Why else would podiatrists offer Botox or surgeons do facelifts on twenty-five-year-olds? I won't do it, and I don't think any of my peers should do it, either.

What I find bizarre about this is the unofficial stance of the American Society of Plastic Surgeons, a conservative organization that positions itself as perched on top of Ethics Mountain for all its members. That's who we surgeons look to for advice about who to treat, and when. So I have been pretty dumbfounded when many of their members have come out and said, "You bet, sure, I would inject filler into someone who is eighteen." That's what I mean about greed.

Finding the Best Plastic Surgeon for You (. . . and What Most of Them Will Never Tell You!)

Any time surgery might be in your future, you have to do your due diligence and make yourself an educated consumer. My advice is to read up on the procedure you're considering, and that's easy enough to do online—but please stick to reputable websites like those of the American Society of Plastic Surgeons, WebMD, or the Mayo Clinic.

Then, make several appointments with surgeons who specialize in the procedure you're considering. Most importantly, you have to know what each procedure can or can't do (which is what this book will teach you). And you have to be prepared to walk out the door if you're being sold something that isn't going to work just so your surgeon can cover his overhead or buy a new car that month. I can always tell who comes to my office prepared. It makes the consultation so much better for both of us.

Read This First So You Don't Get Botched!

Way, *way* too many people assume that plastic surgery is not a big deal because it's elective surgery. But it's still surgery. You will be given anesthesia. You will have some part of your body cut open. You will have things done to muscle, fat, tissues, and skin. You will have stitches. You will bleed.

You will be in pain. You will need prescription pain meds. You will be bruised and look like a truck hit you. You will need time off to recuperate.

In other words, just because you're choosing the procedure doesn't mean that you won't feel bad afterward. Shit happens. You can die.

Here is the "unholy trinity" of how you get botched:

#1: You go to an untrained physician who's maybe taken a weekend course and has very little experience in this procedure.

#2: You're pursuing an unrealistic idea of "perfection." Remember, the enemy of good is better. You need realistic expectations. Plastic surgery can "fix" a body part, but it can't fix your disappointments with life and it can't be seen as a panacea for the emotional, inner work everyone needs to do to find their own happiness.

#3: The luck of the draw. Side effects and complications can happen even though everything was done perfectly. If it only happens to one out of every thousand patients, you certainly do not want to be that one. ***Somebody*** will be!

Every time you have a plastic surgery procedure, and even more so with each subsequent procedure, you're rolling the complication dice and increasing the possibility of longer healing and even more complications. So you think you're not happy (see #2) and want to find a new plastic surgeon and pay him or her to do a touch-up and make it even better? Believe me, you won't have any trouble finding someone to help you out.

Just please do not have an unrealistic view of what can happen, especially about pain and recovery. Even if it's far more common now to get breast augmentation than it was in the past does not mean it's like getting a facial or injectable fillers.

Still want to proceed? Good. An educated patient is a patient who can deal! And your education begins by knowing exactly what to look for in a plastic surgeon and exactly which questions to ask.

Board Certification

If you're going to go to a plastic surgeon, go to a *real* plastic surgeon. You should know that before you walk in the door.

Any licensed medical doctor of any specialty is allowed to perform any medical procedure. Does that mean they should? Of course not. Do you want your obstetrician delivering your baby or injecting your Botox?

In America, surgeons go through four years of medical school, as do all potential doctors, and then have an additional five to nine years of surgical training as interns, residents, and fellows in university training programs. I did six years of general surgery, followed by a fellowship in plastic surgery. I was a board-certified surgeon before I even became a plastic surgeon. After completing a plastic surgery fellowship, a plastic surgeon has to wait two years before even being allowed to take rigorous oral and written testing to obtain certification in plastic surgery. The exams test plastic surgery knowledge, proper technique, and care and avoidance of complications. Also, they need to be repeated every ten years to ensure that surgeons are up to standards and have learned about the newest techniques.

The board certification to look for is by either or both the American Board of Plastic Surgery and the American Board of Facial Plastic and Reconstructive Surgery. For dermatologists, it's the American Board of Dermatology. These are the only boards that are recognized by the American Board of Medical Specialties. Other organizations have "boards" but they are unregulated, and doctors with *these* certifications are not legally allowed to advertise themselves as board certified because these boards are not legally legitimate.

Ask About Operating Privileges

This is one of the most important issues you can bring up. Your surgeon might be board certified, but if he or she doesn't have operating privileges at a local hospital, something is wrong.

Hospitals are an excellent final filter for a surgeon's competence and track record. A surgeon has to apply for them and there is a very thorough vetting, because hospitals don't want anyone in the building who's had a lot of malpractice suits or whose patients have died due to their negligence—or who wants to do what they're not trained to do. So if you don't have hospital privileges, you're either a horrible doctor, or you're not really board certified in what you say you are, such as a dermatologist wanting to do facelifts.

Be wary if your prospective surgeon tries to sell you on the fact he or she has their own surgical suite. Yes, many plastic surgeons do, and it's so much easier to have the procedures done in one place. But it is also a good way to hide the fact that hospital privileges have been denied and a private surgical suite is the only way these surgeons can continue to work.

Look for the Grey Hair

It might come as a bit of a surprise for you to learn that most plastic surgery operations and techniques have remained basically the same for the past twenty years. What's different now is that surgeons do so much *more* of it. I know I was a very good surgeon my first several years in practice— but I have to admit that I was not *that* good. I couldn't possibly have been because I just didn't have the experience.

It's commonly agreed that you need at least ten thousand hours of practice to become truly competent in your field. There isn't a surgeon alive who has that amount of training as a newly minted practitioner; it just isn't physically possible. I was very lucky to have been hired for the TV series *The Swan*, as I had to do so many procedures in a short period of time that it upped my hours working on patients. And ever since *Botched* started and brought me such a wide variety of complicated cases, I know that I am a thousand times better. It's not hubris to say that my volume is so high and I do such incredibly difficult procedures that I sometimes feel almost removed from myself, like watching myself operate now. I'm in the zone, the flow state, the feeling of optimum consciousness, competence, and thinking while I'm doing my work. (And believe me, I am profoundly grateful for these opportunities. It's not that I'm the best; I've just happened to have been given this experience at this moment in my life, and want to do the best I can with what I have to offer.)

But many surgeons, even the best, can only do so much. You can't practice facelifts all day long on real people, but you can train as much as you can as an athlete. Even so, in professional sports, you don't usually get better as you get older, because your body gives out, whereas in occupations like mine—or like aviation, teaching, or acting—you get better the more you do it. Surgeons often say that if they don't operate for a week they can tell the difference, but if they don't operate for two weeks, the *patient* can tell the difference. I know that's true. All surgeons do.

My advice is to avoid using a surgeon who's within five years of graduating. Yes, this might sound harsh, because surgeons need patients in order to improve, but let someone else be the guinea pig. Not you!

You Can Always Find a Surgeon to Do What You Want (. . . and That's Not a Good Thing)

If you go to a surgeon for a consultation and are advised against a certain procedure, it's always smart to get a second or even third opinion. If the next one or two surgeons give you the same advice, perhaps you ought to listen to them.

But I can tell you from years in the business and from all the heinous situations we see on *Botched* that a lot of people do *not* listen. It is really a pathetic indictment of our business where instead of following the spirit of the Hippocratic oath—"First, do no harm"—too many surgeons are in it for the money. Which means you can always, *always*, find someone to do what you want.

You can set yourself up for serious if not lethal complications if you choose to do this, of course. How many times have you read about someone dying after a botched Brazilian butt lift when industrial (and toxic) silicone was mistakenly injected by an unlicensed quack? Or seen photos of someone whose beautiful face was ruined by the wrong kind of fillers or whose nose resembled roadkill after too many procedures? Why would you want to put your body, health, and even life at risk by going to your dentist or gynecologist who took a weekend course to get "certified" in liposuction or filler injection?

Body Dysmorphic Disorder and the Michael Jackson Tragedy

Some of the people we see on *Botched* have body dysmorphic disorder (BDD), which is a rare psychological condition where sufferers become obsessed with a perceived physical defect that, usually, only they can see. They might think their nose is enormous when, in fact, it's perfectly normal. Those with BDD often visit plastic surgeons multiple times to discuss their "flaws," and if they can afford it, they often undergo multiple, unnecessary procedures that usually leave them looking worse.

Plastic surgeons become quite adept at recognizing this disorder, as our sixth sense goes off when the patient doesn't listen, comes back again with a "flaw" that just isn't there, and *still* doesn't listen. I try to never take on these patients, as not only do they need competent psychiatric help, but they're often the first to sue you. Nothing will please them because they have a legitimate mental illness, and surgery is not the answer. Where it gets tricky on *Botched* is when these people with BDD have disabling complications from plastic surgery, yet we still need to find a way to help them; it's one of the most challenging parts of the show.

Michael Jackson often comes up in these discussions. There is no question that he was one of the greatest musical talents of the twentieth century, but he was also one of the most troubled. Allegedly, he had been mocked and tormented by his father about his "big" nose and a typical case of teenage acne, and for his first nose job he went to the best of the best.

I was a medical student when his first nose was done, around the time that *Thriller* was released. One of my brilliant professors at UCLA did it, and it was a gorgeous nose, perfectly shaped and realistic. Michael was happy for a while, but then he went back to the surgeon and asked for more, and the surgeon told him no, absolutely not, don't touch it; once you start messing with it, it's going to get worse. Michael didn't listen and went to another surgeon, who did more nose work and a laundry list of other procedures.

At some point, this became an obsession. It got so bad that sometimes Michael would be put under general anesthesia, *nothing* was done, and then he was bandaged up and told the procedure went well when he woke up. It was a clever, temporary solution to a severe problem—but of course it was also unethical. Michael had gotten to the point where surgeons wanted to work on him to try to fix him, but he was unfixable. And then he died.

I just don't get it. Yes, I know that surgery is very expensive—not just financially but due to the physical toll it takes during the healing process. I get how tempting it is to want to cut corners.

Cosmetic surgery is very rarely a "need" (unless your breasts are painfully large, or your facial expression, such as entrenched frown lines, makes you look like something you're not, which can have a negative effect at your workplace and with loved ones, or there is a genetic abnormality or deformity). Other than those exceptions, cosmetic surgery is a *want*. If it's something you really want, you owe it to yourself and to everyone who cares about you to see an expertly trained and experienced surgeon to help you. Saving your money to pay for the best could save your life.

Know How to Talk to Your Surgeon

To me, the most important thing is your interview with your potential surgeon. Pay attention to two things: How much are they pushing surgery, and are they offering you alternatives? Because if they're not offering you alternatives, you are not going to sign on!

Don't say this: "I really want to have my eyelids done."

Say this instead: "I'm bothered by my eyes. Please tell me what my options are."

See how simple? If you tell the surgeon a surgical option is what you want, that's what you're going to get offered. Instead, you need to hear about all the noninvasive and nonsurgical options, starting with the most economical and least invasive possibilities. So if our patient bothered by her eyes came to me, I'd say, "Let's start with no needles, no nothing. This will actually work if you give it some time and it's going to cost you maybe thirty dollars. The next option is injections, which will cost you three hundred bucks, and it's either not going to work at all or it's going to work really fast."

In other words, I tell my patients how effective each category is, how risky, and how expensive. *That's* a plastic surgeon you should hire. Maybe surgery really is the best option, but it's up to you to find out how many alternatives there are. If you go to several plastic surgeons who have good reputations and they all say the same thing, then check the information in this book and see if it compares.

You also need to be told about potential side effects. If you show a plastic surgeon your breasts because they're a little droopy and he wants to do a lift on you, fine, but he also needs to tell you why a lift might not be good due to scars, side effects, the potential loss of the nipple, and so on. You need all this explained *before* you can give an informed consent. If any risks are brushed aside, say good-bye. You want to hear, "These are your options and these are your risks. Procedure X might be the most effective, but it is surgery, and I have to tell you that some patients with a similar condition have had the nonsurgical Procedure Y and have been just as happy with the results."

That's the best due diligence you can do!

By the way, always consider that maybe you don't need a *perfect* result. If I can give you a 60 percent improvement for $38 with no risks, but it takes six weeks to truly see results, don't you think it's worth a shot? If your surgeon is very busy, you might not be able to have the surgery scheduled for at least six to twelve weeks anyway, so in that case, you've got only $38 to lose and maybe thousands more to save by trying the simplest solution first.

The Slow Month and the Big Cash Flow Factors

Since cosmetic procedures are elective and rarely covered by insurance, making it lucrative for those practitioners who are busy, plastic surgery is a highly competitive field. There are only so many faces to lift and noses to fix.

Let me tell you that even in Beverly Hills or New York City, because there's such a high volume of plastic surgeons, 90 percent of them aren't very busy. Or they're not as busy as they know they can be. Yes, the *crème de la crème* is booked for a year in advance, but if you talk to the average, well-respected surgeon behind closed doors, he's still sweating. He's going, *Fuck, I've got a slow month next month, shit, shit, shit.* Because plastic surgeons are bean counters. We do a case and then we look for another case and another case. Even the best guys are always worried about being slow. So, most of these surgeons are still taking nearly every patient that walks in. Trust me. We all do it!

The Slow Month Factor is important to consider because plastic surgeons tend to be big spenders and have a Big Cash Flow Factor. I can't tell you how many plastic surgeons I know who retire after making a couple of million dollars a year, for decades, with about $500,000 in the bank. They thought the spigot would never stop running and they were not smart about their money. That should never become *your* problem, should it? Of course not.

What does this mean for you, the prospective patient?

For example, if your brow is low but you also have excess upper eyelid skin, doing just your eyelids isn't going to work. You need a forehead lift. But if you tell the surgeon you don't want forehead scars or to pay for a lift, chances are high he's going to agree to your eyelid surgery even though it won't help your descending forehead. It won't *hurt* you—but it won't address the situation. You'll *still* need a brow lift. At least you'll have nice new eyelids and your surgeon will have hit his targets for the week. All the risks and the pros and cons will have been laid out for you, and you will sign off on it. That means your surgeon can operate with a clear conscience. Sort of!

Or, how about just walking out having neither? Or trying Botox instead? So I say, "Look, let's put in a little Botox. It's three hundred bucks, it will only work for three months, and then come back and we'll do some more." They leave happy, and—trust me on this—there isn't a surgeon out there, myself included, who still doesn't think, *Damn, they really need the surgery and I only sold them the Botox.*

So, find the surgeon who might think that way but doesn't *act* on it. The Slow Month Factor has to figure in your due diligence!

Always Ask to See a Lot of Before/After Photos

Plastic surgeons almost always have albums of before/after shots of their patients in their waiting rooms. You really need to look closely at them.

For one thing, this gives you a good assessment of the surgeon's specialty. If there are only two pictures of a facelift and 150 photos of breasts, rest assured that this is a breast guy and not someone for a facelift.

For another, you need to see what kind of technique the surgeon has. A lot of them are known, for example, for doing a certain kind of nose. That might be fabulous for you if this particular nose will look good on your face, but it might be hell for someone else. You want to see a wide range of different noses, and you want to go to someone who's going to give you the right nose for you.

Be sure to look at the photos closely, too. Ideally, the before shot was taken in the same position and lighting as the after shot. It's a big giveaway if the before photo is poorly lit and with a scowling patient, and the patient looks happy and is perfectly composed and lit in the after shot. Also be wary if the before shot shows a bare face and the face in the after shot is beautifully made up. That's a fail!

Ask About the Anesthesia

Many surgeons use nurse anesthetists, who are highly trained and can be very good. But I don't want to be the only person in charge of the entire room, including anesthesia, which is, after all, what puts you in a chemical coma. If there's an emergency and everything's going to shit, if you're using a nurse anesthetist you only have one doctor in the room. If you have an anesthesiologist, you now have two doctors, including the anesthesia expert. (The medical school joke is that anesthesia is 99 percent boredom and 1 percent sheer terror.) Honestly, what do I know about it? I know a *bit*, but I can't even turn the machines on and off. I don't use them. I trust the anesthesiologist to use them.

In other words, I drive a Porsche. I don't know how to *fix* the Porsche. I don't *want* to know, either. I just want to do my job to the best of my abilities and surround myself with the best, most highly trained specialists to help me. That means an MD anesthesiologist who did a five-year anesthesia residency. It's the same reason why you'd rather have a SWAT officer protect you in a home invasion than the security guy from some company down the street.

I sincerely doubt that any harm will come to you if your surgeon of choice uses an excellent nurse anesthetist. But just be sure to ask, because you have the right to know!

Ask About Risks

Always, always ask about risks. I have patients who come in, all flustered and anxious to get the procedure done because a wedding is coming up, or summer's going to be here soon, or they just got invited to an important event and they need to be on the table now, now, *now*!

That is not how you plan your surgery.

You don't want your doctor to have a cavalier attitude about risks and be all friendly and sales-pitchy. Surgery is surgery, whether elective or lifesaving. Chances are slim, but it can always have catastrophic results.

121

I'd estimate that some procedures almost never have complications, some have complications 5 percent to 10 percent of the time, and some are extremely risky. A body lift after massive weight loss has a 30 percent chance of having a complication. That means there will be a problem with one out of three procedures. Do these patients know the risks and still want to go ahead? Almost always, yes, because there is no other way to get rid of the excess skin.

If your surgeon downplays the risks, that's not the doctor for you because they're not being honest. Even the very best doctors have all experienced the worst complications during surgeries. This has nothing to do with their skill level—it's just bad luck. (One of the worst kinds of bad luck is picking up an infection in a hospital after surgery—it has nothing to do with the procedure and happens incredibly often.) Think of it this way: Even world-class racecar drivers have totaled their cars. They know what they're doing. But sometimes there's an oil slick on the road and the car spins out of control and they're done for—due solely to bad luck.

I tell every patient, "I need to talk to you about the risks." They nod. I go, "Do you know what the worst thing is that can happen to you with this breast augmentation?" They ask, and I reply, "You can get a blood clot in your leg. If it breaks off and goes to your lung, it's called a pulmonary embolism and you can die."

Usually, this is followed by paled cheeks and a shocked look in their eyes.

But, to be perfectly honest here, it is also a reverse sales technique that is very clever. Because I am being candid and truthful, I am also making my patients think, *Wow, this guy is so honest!* I want him to do my surgery. So it's a win/win. I have the work I want to do, and the patient has confidence in me.

Your surgeon should be this honest, too. Ask if he or she has ever encountered any severe complications during surgeries. I've had seven pulmonary embolisms in my career but I haven't had any deaths because I'm so paranoid about it. I know what to look out for and I tell my patients that at the first sign of shortness of breath, I'm sending them right to the ER. I'm also instructing them to tell the ER triage that they need a spiral CT, an X-ray designed to quickly diagnose pulmonary embolism, because Terry Dubrow is worried about it. If you catch it, no biggie. You'll spend maybe two days in the hospital, and then you'll be fine.

In fact, I am so paranoid about this that I can sometimes diagnose complications when they're not even there yet. I get a weird Spidey sense when it might happen—I can't explain why. Most really good surgeons I know have the same premonitions. We can *feel* it. I don't know if "spiritual" is the right word for it; it's more of a psychic vibe. I think that everyone who's really good at their jobs has a sixth sense. You could be a billionaire CEO who backs out of seemingly solid deal or a construction guy who gets a bad feeling at work one day and refuses to go up in the elevator, only to see it crash an hour later.

This is why surgeons should never mind being asked about the risks!

Ask About Pain

As I wrote earlier in this chapter, the pain factor of surgery is often grossly underestimated by many patients, who think they're going to wake up after the procedure, maybe need a Tylenol or two, stay in bed for a day, and go on their merry way. Sorry, but that is *never* going to happen!

If you're having a breast augmentation, the muscles in and around your very sensitive breasts are going to be moved. If you have a tummy tuck, the muscles of your core are going to be cut, tightened, and sewn back up. Think about it. Every time you breathe and move, your core muscles are affected. Having any kind of insult to them is going to hurt like hell.

Some people are naturally more pain-tolerant than others. Some can't cope at all. Some have trouble with the side effects of pain medication; in the worst-case scenario, others become addicted to their pain meds and their lives turn into nightmares.

Please, be realistic about your pain tolerance and discuss it candidly with your surgeon. If you've ever had any problems with certain meds, now

Never, Ever Lie to Your Surgeon

One of the biggest risks is when patients aren't up front about any health issues.

Highest on that list is smoking. I can usually tell the chronic smokers because their clothes tend to be permeated by smoke, no matter how much perfume has been used or gum is being chewed. I usually also see a brief look of panic when I ask about any smoking habits.

The reason smoking is so dangerous for surgery is because the nicotine literally cuts off and reduces the flow of blood to the soft tissues and the skin. If you reduce the blood supply to the tissues and skin, it can lead to poor oxygen delivery and cell death, which can lead to skin death called necrosis. It's a horrible complication that will cause terrible scarring, distortion of the treated area, and possibly serious infections. At the very least, smoking can prolong your recuperation and make complications more likely.

Another common lie I've been told is when someone says they never had a nose job before and then when I opened them up, there was scarring and lack of healthy tissue. It may not seem like a little fib, but it could have been a major problem. Even worse are those patients who leave out important pieces of medical information because they are either embarrassed or worried I will cancel their surgery. For example, I had a patient omit her history of recently diagnosed heart disease, knowing I would not have agreed to operate, and she suffered a very scary but ultimately fixable cardiac problem. I have had patients who, despite orders to stop two weeks earlier, take aspirin right before surgery, deny doing so, and bleed significantly during and after an operation due to the anticlotting effects of aspirin. My favorite is when patients deny having any facial surgeries and then, when asked about the facial scars, say, "Oh, that? I just had a little chin lift."

Bottom line: An experienced surgeon is going to have a pretty good idea if you're not telling the truth. Don't let that be you!

is not the time to be shy. Speak up. Most patients do well after surgery, take the meds they need, and throw out the rest. But if the postoperative pain is unrelenting, something is wrong. Call your surgeon right away!

Ask About Postoperative Care

It's very important to ask about postoperative care, because that is when you are most vulnerable and when many minor complications become major ones.

Ask who does your post-op care—is it your surgeon or a physician's assistant or a nurse? Not that these practitioners aren't competent and well trained; some patients really don't care who sees them, while others would be very upset if the surgeon didn't do the follow-up.

Also, who will you talk to if you have questions or problems after office hours? I always give my patients my cell phone number after their surgeries and tell them they can call me 24/7. It can be a double-edged sword, because they can call at all hours, but it's still worth it, as small problems treated immediately remain small problems. My patients know that if they can always get ahold of me, they relax and feel safe. They also can't sue me—which, unfortunately, is something that all surgeons have to think about all the time.

Before I started doing this, we would always get the Friday-night-at-eight panicking phone calls because these patients freaked, worrying that they wouldn't be able to get any help over the weekend. Inevitably, when I asked what the issue was and how long they'd had it, they would tell me four days. They'd ignored it all week! Giving out my cell phone number has completely taken all of that worry away.

Bedside Manner Matters

There are many jokes and assumptions made about a surgeon's personality —or alleged lack thereof!—and it is true that the person cutting you open doesn't necessarily have to have the trusting, winning personality of someone you'll be seeing on a more regular basis for your health care, such as your primary physician.

But bedside manner is still very important. Plastic surgeons tend to be more engaging than other specialists, as we know our procedures are elective. You're not going to hire us if we're not friendly and welcoming. Still, be smart and be skeptical. Behind that kind, wide smile might be a very cleverly constructed sales pitch!

Another trait that is very important to consider is *confidence*. Obviously, you want your surgeon to be well versed in the latest techniques and highly experienced. But you also don't want your surgeon to be so over-confident and such an egomaniac that preventable blunders are going to be made—at *your* expense.

I have plenty of peers who are extremely talented surgeons but who have much higher than normal complication rates. I was very fortunate to have been trained in general surgery, so no matter what I'm doing, I go through my paranoia-that-something-can-go-wrong checklist to ensure that nothing *does* go wrong. I don't let the fact that I'm good at my job interfere with how I do it. *No one* is immune to mistakes. Real confidence shines through when surgeons are honest about the realities of surgery, its pros and cons, their experience, and how they act if and when things go wrong. That is the kind of confidence I want to see in a person holding a scalpel over my skin.

Ask About Lawsuits

Anyone can sue anybody for anything. America is the most litigious country in the world, and just because someone has pending lawsuits doesn't make them a bad doctor. What counts are *judgments* and *settlements*. A settlement is when you agree to pay the patient in order to settle a problem you had with their care and treatment. A judgment is a verdict in court that says a judge or jury has concluded that the surgical care was negligent and below the acceptable standards of care.

Substantial settlements are significant, because it means the surgeon did wrong and knows he or she is going to lose the case. A small settlement, not as much, because surgeons often will return a patient's fees or even settle for a small amount to avoid the painful and time-consuming process of a medical malpractice trial.

In plastic surgery, I'd estimate that 98 percent of malpractice lawsuits are totally frivolous. Far too often, surgeons are sued simply because the patients don't want to pay. It's as simple as that—a high-profile shakedown—and surgeons have been known to settle just to save on legal fees and make these jerks go away. Of course, it's greedy patients like that who cause prices to go up for everyone else.

Once, I did a breast reduction, a tummy tuck, and facial work on a patient. I killed it with some of my best results ever. All I did was be honest—I wrote down exactly how much tissue I took out of her breasts and the insurance company claimed that it wasn't enough for her to meet the criteria for reimbursement. She was so pissed that she sued me for malpractice with the boilerplate complaint: "practicing below the standard of care." Believe me, if this had been malpractice, I would have been the first to admit it. But it was an insurance shakedown. When it became clear I wouldn't roll over, she quickly dismissed the case for fear of being sued for malicious prosecution.

Fortunately, medical malpractice isn't such a big deal in California as it is in other states. We have a law known as MICRA, for Medical Injury Compensation Reform Act, which states that if you are maimed but can still earn a living, or even if you die, then the maximum damages payout for pain and suffering is $250,000. This is scant consolation to the family of someone who died due to a botched procedure, but it does cut way down on frivolous lawsuits because it's impossible to get a big payout. Only the bottom-feeder lawyers here bother with it.

Don't Pay Attention to Media or Hype

When it comes to evaluating a surgeon's credentials and record, social media is pretty much worthless. So are patient reviews. So are bad plastic surgery websites. So are celebrity photos on the walls of the surgeon's waiting room.

For example, I have thousands of good reviews on Yelp, but due to the filtering process, it's not always easy to find them. I can tell you that the handful of really bad reviews are bogus ones put up by some of my competition. Yes, it really is that petty—and yes, this makes all reviews pretty much worthless if you can't tell which are real and which are bogus. I know that a lot of surgeons hate me because I'm on *Botched*. (They feel the same about my partner, Paul; we don't take professional jealousy personally.) But I take my work very seriously

As for websites, mine is pretty bare bones. I give basic information on some of my most popular procedures, but it's not how I need to sell myself. In fact, I think that the fanciest websites are often smokescreens for less-than-genius surgeons. It's nice to see a super-fancy or slick design, but it shouldn't be a selling point. Photos can easily be Photoshopped. Testimonials can be invented.

You already know that you should do your own research on sites not affiliated with any particular practitioner. What really counts is what's discussed during your consultations.

As for patient referrals, unless they're your friends, patients who volunteer information about their surgeon are rarely going to tell you the unvarnished truth. You're just not going to be able to find out if the recommendation is unsolicited or not. So don't use a surgeon's willingness to give you names as something that will truly be helpful in making an accurate assessment.

Then there are the websites devoted to assessing bad or botched plastic surgery. I know that scanning them is a guilty pleasure, but a lot of my patients think the information is accurate because it was allegedly written by a real plastic surgeon. But here's the catch—the actual surgeon who performed the procedures is the *only* one truly qualified to comment. Instead, the website surgeons are pontificating about something they only saw in photographs. It's all based on bullshit they don't really know.

Why? Well, I have news for you. You can take any of my patients three days out from a procedure and they all look like shit. For example, I once injected a long-time patient and something funky happened to her forehead. The veins were popping out and she looked like a Klingon. She freaked and called me all sorts of names, including "the worst plastic surgeon in the world," and I calmly told her I understood why she was upset, to ice it, and to stop worrying. (I wasn't worried, even though her husband is a malpractice attorney!) I promised her it would go away and it did, after a few more weeks. Several months later she returned for more injections, and we both had a good laugh. But if someone had taken before/after photos while this situation was going on, I would have been severely judged and she would have considered herself botched.

One last thing: I tell celebrities not to come to me, and for several good reasons. They want everything for free. They think they're entitled and I should drop everything to cater to them. They want me to come to their house. And if my work on them goes right they tell no one and if it goes wrong they tell everyone. What's the point? The risk and the aggravation outweigh the benefits for me.

Celebrity clients are more understandable for a younger, up-and-coming surgeon trying to build up a client base. But I still would not be happy if I were a patient and I walked into an office and saw lots of celebrity photos. You can't help but wonder if the surgeon is a star-fucker who'll give preferential care to the celebrities. All patients are equal, at least to me!

Getting Personal Recommendations from Your Friends Isn't Enough

Heather and I find it incredible that people planning to buy a car will shop for months and compare prices and read the professional buyers report, too. They know how important it is to do due diligence for such a big purchase. But with plastic surgery, they say, "Oh my friend had her boobs done by so-and-so and they look good." And that's enough for them to sign right up.

Believe me, that is *not* enough!

Heather has several friends who listened to one person, who assured them how fabulous a particular Beverly Hills surgeon was. All these friends went to him, and they had a complication. They didn't check to see what his status was with the medical board or look at any of his patient before/after photos or ask him any questions. Don't let this happen to you.

Yes, Some Patients Are Beyond *Help—and I Can't Give Them the Results They Actually Need*

Once, a patient said, "I want this, and I want that, and I want you to do it next week, and you are going to do this . . ." I looked at her in disbelief because she was so unbelievably unpleasant and it made me almost hate her. I excused myself and walked out, handed her chart to my office manager, and said, "I'm not working on this person. *Not for a million dollars!*" Then I turned around and found the patient standing there, glaring at me. "Okay, smart-ass," she said. "How about $58,000?"

"Great," I replied. "I'll do it."

That's a *joke*, by the way!

Seriously, though, I've had some patients ask for some crazy things over the years. On *Botched*, we get asked to do breast implants on men and put plastic hearts under the skin—but in my regular practice I've been asked to do much weirder things. One man asked for devil horns on his head; another asked for breast implants on his *back* after he lost a poker bet.

The best plastic surgeons become adept at listening to our patients so we can assess their psychological needs. Do they want a nose job because they have a big nose, or because they think it's preventing them from finding a husband or wife? Does that woman with perfectly lovely C-cup breasts ask for implants because she genuinely wants them or because her boyfriend threatened to leave if she didn't go through with it? Does the fifty-year-old who's already had two facelifts need another one, or is she looking for something she'll never find?

I've found that the patients who are very angry or disappointed with life sometimes try to transfer their unhappiness to me. Most of the time I realize who they are preoperatively and gently turn them away, because their problems are psychological, not physical, and they need competent counseling for their mental health issues more than they need surgery. Although, of course, they can always find someone to do what they want.

I wish more of my colleagues were able to say no to someone who is clearly in trouble, if not diagnosable mentally ill.

Sometimes, though, those with psychological issues are extremely clever at masking them, and they pass my initial filtering mechanism and red flag detection and I take them on. They're rarely satisfied even with the most stunning results, whine about every single aspect of healing, come in for endless appointments and complain some more, and often extort you to the point where you want to pay them off just to go away and torment another surgeon.

I don't think it's so much a case of body dysmorphic disorder as it is a void in their lives that they think surgery will magically fix. But, as you well know, making external changes can't do anything if you don't make internal changes at the same time. Plastic surgery can make you look so much better and hopefully in doing so will improve your confidence level in your appearance. And that's it. Expecting more is unrealistic and setting yourself up for disappointment.

It's a challenge to postoperatively recommend a patient seek psychological help, because they often see that as the doctor wanting to dismiss them and their complaints as just being "crazy." At the end of the day, many plastic surgery patients, like everyone, have emotional and psychological issues that could be worked on, but once a surgical procedure is involved, it can make the situation dramatically worse or bring all the deeper issues suddenly to the surface. Please, if you're considering surgery, look deeply inside yourself and make sure you have realistic goals and expectations and you're doing it for the right reason.

Last but Not Least . . . Always Trust Your Gut

Remember how I talked about my Spidey sense of feeling that something might go wrong with a patient? I am so tuned in to what I need to do when they're on the table that all my senses are on fire. They're also highly attuned when a potential patient comes in and is a little . . . off.

You need to trust your gut, too. Do your due diligence and take your time to find the right surgeon. If you're at your consultation and your sixth sense starts pinging, get up and leave. No apologies needed. I don't care if this person has been recommended to you as the best in the world—if you're not feeling it *prior* to surgery, you certainly won't feel it *afterward*. You have to like your plastic surgeon. You have to have the utmost confidence in him or her. Take a pause and reevaluate later. It's elective surgery; it's not an urgent or emergency situation. It may ultimately be the right procedure with the right doctor but just not at that time. That internal voice, I have found, is usually extremely accurate.

One caveat, however: once you decide to get a procedure done, let yourself go. Go in with a great attitude and expect a good outcome. This kind of positive thinking will allow your mind and body to heal to the best of its ability and can make the difference between a problematic outcome and a great result.

Heather—On Esthetics, Critics, and Making Sure You Really Need Plastic Surgery

Do you remember the TV cartoon show *The Jetsons*? The mom's name was Jane, and she put what she called her morning mask on—which was so funny to me, because when I was a kid, my mom would say, "Oh, I can't go out until I put my face on," meaning her makeup. *Jane's* version was an actual mask so that when anyone called her on the videophone she looked all done up. Imagine that! A videophone! That was considered the height of future chic—and now look at us. We're always online, on Skype or Face-Time, sometimes at the most inopportune time, and Jane Jetson's cartoon fantasy has become our daily reality.

If you're a Hollywood performer and wife of a well-known plastic surgeon as I am, you realize the critics are out there lurking, waiting to pounce on you with comments about aging, about treatments, about distorted images in the media, about self-worth as judged by the lines (or lack thereof) on our faces. Sometimes the swift and stabbing judgments make me want to vomit. I won't bend over at the beach or pool because I've had four kids and no matter how much I work out, there is extra skin and I'm worried about being caught on film at the wrong angle and ending up in the "Worst Beach Bodies" issue of *Star* magazine! So, I understand the need or desire to have things fixed or tweaked . . . but when is enough enough?

I think that one of the reasons the awful plastic surgery websites are so popular is they spot people who do keep going and going so that they're absolutely unrecognizable. And then whoever it is in the spotlight becomes known for *that*. I'm of the opinion that everyone wants to be famous. Not necessarily famous on television, but famous for something special, to have that validation. It could be that you make the best casserole, or throw the best parties in town, or write the best articles, or have the biggest lips in your state. The fact that, for some people, the external is their only validation makes me so sad, because we all know at the end of the day, your true validation is based on who you are inside and what you do in this lifetime, not what you look like. I mean, who wants to be in the *Guinness Book of World Records* for having enormous boobs? Apparently quite a few people, since this is actually a category that exists! *Yikes!*

Often, the critics who go after me and other celebrities say, "Oh, I would *never* have plastic surgery," but they'll color their hair and get Botox and filler and laser hair removal. Many of them are still very young, and they don't realize that their thinking might shift as they grow older and start living with much more noticeable changes. It's sort of like the people who swear they'd never yell at their kids . . . until they have kids! We all think we are going to be perfect parents (so different than *our* parents . . .) until the first time our precious little darlings have a full-on screaming tantrum in the middle of the grocery store and we totally lose it!

So, where is the line drawn? And why does anyone care where everyone's line is, anyway? Everyone's line is different. Maybe you and your husband are vegetarians, but he will eat fish if it's served at someone else's home. Or you don't wear fur. Okay, so you won't wear fur, but you'll wear leather. See what I mean? There are a thousand different shades of grey.

I also think that you can't blame Hollywood people for their seemingly endless attention to their appearance, because part of being a Hollywood star is to be forever youthful, to retain a sort of unattainable beauty that's almost unworldly. But because that is unattainable for most people, there's a lot of nitpicking and criticism, perhaps so we can feel a little better about ourselves when we find flaws in seemingly "flawless" stars.

It's the same reason people want to watch reality television about celebrities. Sure, it's partly aspirational, because who doesn't want to be free from money worries and have mansions and take private jets? But it's also human nature to want to see those who seemingly have it all deal with the same daily ups and downs and craziness of life.

The most important thing is to be comfortable with who you are and how you look. I've seen people around town that try to pretend they haven't had any work done when their butts are the size of a Goodyear blimp. I've also talked to hundreds of people who are happily honest about what they've had done and eager to keep up with the latest technology and procedures.

It all goes back to what I said about experimenting first. I'm talking about your body. It's really important. You only have one. Having surgery is not like trying on a new lipstick or getting a piercing or getting your hair dyed. I see so many people going for trendy treatments like the Brazilian butt lift that they may regret in a short few years. Following trends because people you like are falling for them and not thinking through the results is often a recipe for disaster. You don't need to watch an episode of *Botched* to know that! I'm especially concerned lately about the all-too-popular "Mommy Makeover" that many women seem to run to get six months to two years after their last child. I will tell you from my own experience that, yes, your body changes after each pregnancy; now, however, five years after having my last child, I'm *amazed* how my body has bounced back! I didn't think it was possible, but diet and exercise and just maybe time did the trick?

What I'm getting to is that, of course, I'm a proponent of plastic surgery, but only in the right setting, on the right body part, with the right surgeon, and when it's done for the right reason. If your nose has always bothered you and a change is going to enhance your life, do it. Do anything that's going to make you feel good, but not with a spur-of-the-moment decision and not without answering all of these questions on this checklist.

Heather's Presurgery Checklist

You know how sometimes someone gets you so mad or hurt that you fire off an angry e-mail—and then regret it the minute you hit "Send" and can't take it back? Well, when I'm in that kind of state, I write that enraged e-mail and send it to *myself*. I don't want to do anything when I'm not thinking clearly that I might feel terrible about later.

This checklist is the equivalent of the e-mail to yourself, except it's about plastic surgery. It's my emotional list that will go along with all the information Terry has already given you, as well as the medical list your surgeon will give you. You know, the one that tells you to stop smoking and get off Advil, and about any possible complications. Take your time with this. If you're sure of your answers, then you're ready to do it. Here's what to ask yourself:

❖ Am I in the best possible health now so I can realistically assess my body's shape? For example, am I desperate for a Mommy Makeover to get my boobs and belly done, but my body is still recuperating from the birth of my last child? In my case, I used to have large natural breasts . . . then I had four kids and these lovely breasts went away. That's what happens; your body changes. For a hot second I thought about getting them done, and then I thought, number one, I have a latex allergy and with my luck I'd have severe complications, and number two, it seemed way too cliché to be married to a plastic surgeon, living in Orange County, and having fake boobs. I just couldn't do it. And then, weirdly, what's happened over the years is that my breasts have totally grown back. Not to what they once were, but I'm not complaining! Sure, implants and a lift would have given me shape and upper fullness, but the point is sometimes you have to let your body sit for months if not years so you can then make a more accurate assessment about areas that are bothering you.

❖ Have I done everything possible with my regular exercise routine yet still have problem areas? For example, liposuction is for thin or normal-weight people; it's not for weight loss, only pockets of stubborn fat that don't go away no matter how much you exercise. If that's not me, am I willing to take however long it needs to get myself in the best possible health and shape and only then make an informed decision about what I've been able to accomplish on my own?

❖ Am I totally certain I can live with a permanent alteration of the looks I've had all my life? That's always scared me. Everyone thinks I've had my nose done, but I haven't. Trust me, I would have had it done in high school, but I didn't need it done. I like my nose! Sure, sometimes I still look at that bump on one side and wonder if it's getting wider with age, but then I think, wow, would I rather risk having one of those nose-job-looking noses that I'd have to look at every day for the rest of my life, or live with this? I think you know the answer!

❖ Am I judging myself against somebody else? Am I falling into the competition trap? You have to figure out what is the real you that you want to enhance as opposed to change. Honestly, this is something I totally understand. Last year, I posted a bikini photo on social media. I usually never do this sort of thing, but we were in Hawaii and I was really proud of myself because I'd been working out a lot. Now, to be clear, I didn't show my butt or my cellulite! There were a lot of nice comments, but there were also a lot of comments saying I looked like that only because my husband's a plastic surgeon. Excuse me? What did he do? Was he in the gym doing my sit-ups and squats for me? All I had done is Botox and Sculptra, and only in my face—nowhere else. I still have to work out regularly and watch what I eat. It's hard. Often, it's frustrating. It takes a lot of time. And it's crazy that people would just automatically assume I've had everything done just because, theoretically, I could.

On social media, people post an idealized version of what they want you to think about them—a.k.a. my "ideal" life on Instagram—and you can't help but judge yourself against that. It really bothers me, and yet even I did it once, when I took the kids to a theme park and we had a terrible time. They acted up and were awful, and I posted a Happy Family picture anyway. I felt so *phony*. I'm never doing that again!

❖ *Am I worrying about what I'll look like at some point in the future instead of dealing with the now?* It's crazy but I think we all, to some degree, are super critical of our bodies. I have to admit that sometimes, when I put on a bikini, I think I can't go out in it for fear someone might take my photo and post it online to make me cry. If I mention that to Terry, he'll say, "I wish you could be happy with how fantastic you look like now, because if you *could* see what you might look like ten or twenty years from now, you would wish you had *this* body back!" How can you argue with that?

❖ *Am I convinced that if I have plastic surgery, my life will magically change?* Do I think that if I fix this one thing, the rest of my life will fall into place? If so, I think you need to sit down, reassess your goals, and do the internal work about what is good/bad/lacking in your life, and then come up with more tangible and realistic ways to attain those goals before you do something permanent that you might regret. Especially if the magical change doesn't materialize.

❖ *Am I doing my best to make myself happy?* It might sound trite, but when you're super happy with who you are and where you are in your life, you look happy and you look beautiful and you look *young*. The best way to keep yourself youthful is to be a good person and be generous, because then it's given back to you. Happiness is contagious, after all. It's why we love weddings so much, and why brides can be literally transformed on their wedding day.

Every day, you should do something that makes you happy. Terry and I will send each other Buddhist quotes. They make me feel good and put a smile on my face. I know people who find a few minutes of inspirational happiness looking at cat videos or soldiers-coming-home videos during their breaks at work. Or things that make them laugh, because laughter makes them happy. (One of my favorites is an Instagram page called Asshole Parents. It kills me every time, and makes me realize that I'm not such a bad mommy even if my temper-tantrum-prone five-year-old would beg to differ!) Every morning, when I take the kids to school, we put our pointer fingers to our foreheads like a unicorn point. It's our secret signal to each other in honor of the mystical creatures. It makes us happy. It makes me look better. And then I'm ready to face the rest of the day with a smile on my face.

❖ *Last but not least, am I clear in understanding that perfection doesn't exist?* Perfection is nothing more than a perfect version of *you*. That's all!

Terry Tips for the Best Way to Recuperate After Surgery

Surgery is always a shock to the body, even for minor procedures, and you need to give yourself time to recuperate. The enemy of good healing is impatience! Here are my tips to make the process as safe and smooth as possible:

❖ Call your surgeon if you have any questions. Don't ignore anything you think might be wrong. Better to be safe than sorry!

One thing to watch out for is your heart rate. If your resting pulse goes over 100, I expect you to be calling me immediately. If your pulse is that high and you suddenly get very thirsty, that is a life-threatening emergency. Call 911 and get to the ER *stat*. I'll tell you why: When I was the chief resident of general surgery at UCLA, two brothers came in after stupidly getting into a fight and stabbing each other. The older brother got stabbed three times in his belly by the younger brother; the younger brother got stabbed once in the lower chest by the older brother. Did I say stupid? Anyway the trauma team is getting ready while the brothers are cursing each other (and us) out. We know the older brother has intestinal holes and maybe a liver injury. All of a sudden the younger brother goes, "I'm thirsty." Well, I knew that's a really bad sign, because if your pulse is elevated and you're breathing so fast that you haven't passed out yet, there's some signal in your brain that activates the thirst center. I said, "You're thirsty?" He said, "Yeah." Without hesitation, I put him under, cracked his chest open, saw the hole in his heart, put in two stitches, closed it up, closed *him* up, and he walked out of the hospital ten days later. He found me in the cafeteria and thanked me. He would have been dead literally one minute later, and everyone had told him I saved his ass.

So why am I telling you this? It's not because you'll be getting stabbed in the heart by your crazy older brother. It's because *you have to listen to your body*. If something is off, there is a reason for it. It could be the most benign reason that is just a normal part of healing. Or not. Take your healing seriously!

❖ Follow instructions. If you are told to wear a compression garment, wear it. If you're told to sleep with your head elevated, don't lie on your side. If you're told no showers, use extra deodorant. You can cause serious complications if you don't do exactly as you are told.

❖ Stay clean. After surgery, your incision sites will be properly bandaged. It's imperative to keep the wounds clean to promote healing and prevent infections. Always follow your surgeon's directions about changing the bandages, especially if there are drains to help get rid of fluids.

❖ Eat smart. What you want to eat are fresh, whole foods—especially vegetables, whole grains, fruit, and lean proteins like chicken and fish—that provide essential nutrients to aid in healing. Avoid all junk foods, anything packaged or fake, and anything high in salt and saturated fat. These crummy foods can cause inflammation and bloating, which can delay the healing process.

❖ Rest—but not too much! Getting plenty of rest is a must, especially the first few days after surgery. But you need to get up and get gently walking around as soon as you are able to. This gets your blood circulating, which encourages tissues to heal more quickly.

❖ Ease back into your exercise routine. Follow your surgeon's instructions about when to resume aerobic activities or going to the gym. Even professional athletes need time to heal, and they're often terrible about listening to me because they're always on the move. Pace yourself! Start slow. If you go at it too hard, you might find yourself back on restricted activities and have to start the waiting process all over again.

❖ Don't even think about smoking. It will definitely make healing a lot more difficult because it constricts blood flow. As I told you already, never, ever lie to your surgeon about your smoking. I insist that my patients who smoke cut it out completely for at least four weeks prior to and after surgery. I know how hard this can be, but I'm not about to endanger someone's life for a cosmetic procedure because they're addicted!

❖ Believe in the placebo effect. The placebo effect is very real and very powerful. It's an important adjunct to how I work with my patients—because so much of what comprises healing goes on in your head just as it does in your body. If, for example, I tell my patients that they are healing so much faster that everyone else, they actually do heal so much faster. The placebo effect is really all about the power of positive thinking.

Here's something you might not know. You are probably aware that the over-prescription of antibiotics is leading to the development of antibiotic-resistant bacteria, which is a terrifying thought. But for most plastic surgery procedures, you only need to be given one dose of intravenous antibiotics preoperatively, within an hour of the surgical cut time. If the procedure is "clean," we aren't supposed to give patients postoperative oral antibiotics; they don't really need them. But we always do it anyway, for two reasons. One is because if we don't and there's a complication, the patient will be more likely to engage in a malpractice lawsuit. The second is that patients wonder why you didn't, since they've always been prescribed antibiotics after surgery before. The result? The chances that they'll actually get an infection go *up* due to the placebo effect!

If, on the other hand, a patient really is starting to get red around their incision, I'm a little concerned about infection. I prescribe the antibiotic, but I also harness the power of the placebo effect by telling them it's one of the most effective and incredible drugs out there, and they take it right away and the worry is gone. Was it a super-drug? No—it was merely an effective broad-spectrum antibiotic. But it was a super-drug for their *brain*.

If any organ can truly help you with the healing process, it's your brain. You can psyche yourself up for anything. You can will yourself to heal more quickly. You can be confident and loving toward the incredible body you live in. You can focus on the positive, even if you do get a complication.

Focus on the negative, however, and I can promise you that you'll hurt more and take longer to heal.

For example, take me right now. Literally, I get up at four in the morning and operate until six every night, I'm more successful than I've ever been and having a better time than I've had in my entire life, even though I'm massively sleep deprived. My family's great, everything's great, but I'm working harder than ever. You give me the exact same hours, make me do the exact same thing and don't give me any money, don't put me on television, don't give me any great feedback . . . and I guarantee you that I will look much older, much greyer, much more wrinkled, and just blah all over. But because I'm happy I don't look as bad as I should look right now; with my punishing schedule, I should look like death warmed over. That I don't is due not to my skincare regimen (although that helps!) but my *brain*. I make my own placebo effect. And it sure feels good!

◇◇◇◇◇◇◇◇◇◇◇◇◇◇◇◇◇◇◇◇◇◇

Now that you know what to look for if you're considering plastic surgery, turn to the next chapter for details about the best anti-aging procedures.

CHAPTER

7

Plastic Surgery Procedures

You're ready to go, right? The time has arrived. You want to look your best, only more youthful, and these are the most sought-after surgeries that can help you turn back the clock.

I haven't included all the surgeries I do—for example, chin implants are often done with nose jobs, but that's more of an esthetic decision to balance facial proportions and won't change the aging factor; and neck lifts are only recommended for men, as they can create a jarring contrast of skin texture between neck and face. These and other procedures don't relate to anti-aging, but I list the most common ones that do, and that will give you visible results.

Note: The pain meter is rated on a scale of 1 to 10, with 1 being nearly painless and 10 being screaming for mercy. This scale is based on the ability to control the pain with medication, and the type and strength of the pain medications required to control the pain. For example 1–3 pain is easily controlled with a short-term course of Tylenol or Advil; 4–7 pain requires a narcotic-type medication like Vicodin or Tylenol with codeine; 7 and above would require a high-level narcotic like Percocet or even a short-term injectable like morphine or Demerol.

Plastic Surgery Procedures—Head and Neck

Eyes—Upper and Lower Blepharoplasty

I love seeing women with laugh lines around their eyes. Forget calling them crow's feet or wrinkles—they're signs of people enjoying their lives and not afraid to show it. But, sometimes, especially due to the natural laxity of the tender and vulnerable skin of the eye area, help is needed. Drooping or saggy eyelids can make you look a lot older and more exhausted than you really are—and sometimes can even affect your vision—and there is a simple procedure to correct this.

What It Does

Blepharoplasty, or eyelid surgery, can repair sagging upper eyelids, drooping lower eyelids, excess fat deposits that make the eyelids puffy, and wrinkles around the eye area.

How It's Done

This surgery is done under either local or general anesthesia. For an upper blepharoplasty, an incision is made in the natural fold of the upper eyelid where excess skin and fat deposits are removed. After the upper eyelid muscles are repositioned, the incision is closed. For a lower blepharoplasty, an incision is made just below the lash line to remove excess skin and fat. In most instances, another incision is placed inside of the lower eyelid to diminish puffiness under the eyes. Once the lower eyelid muscles are repositioned, the incisions are closed. Because all of the incisions are made inconspicuously in the eyelids, you won't have to worry about noticeable scars.

Realistic Expectations

It takes about one to two weeks for the swelling to go down completely so you can see the final results. If your surgeon was smart and removed and tightened the right amount of skin, your eyes will appear larger and smoother, but not jarringly different. You will simply look well rested and more youthful.

Pain Meter

1–2. Pain is usually minimal and if you take your pain medication and use cold compresses, it will help with discomfort and swelling.

Recuperation Time

About a week—you should be able to return to work then. Be sure to use sunglasses and sunscreen in the area, and stay out of the sun or bright light so you don't strain your eyes and want to rub them. Avoid any strenuous activities for at least two weeks.

Possible Complications/What Can Go Wrong

Although a seemingly simple procedure, a blepharoplasty can lead to significant problems if not done correctly or if the doctor didn't evaluate the anatomy properly. The best thing to do is, while looking in the mirror, pull down and release your lower eyelid. If the "snap-back" seems slow when you let go, you are at risk of the lower eyelid skin healing in a pulled-down, basset-hound appearance. If the snap-back is delayed, you *must* also have a corner-tightening procedure to prevent the postoperative pull-down. Always do this test and discuss the results with your surgeon!

As for esthetics, when too much skin is removed, patients look unnatural and unlike themselves. You don't want people to do a double take—your eyes are the first thing people notice about your face and believe me, you don't want any extreme changes. If too much upper eyelid skin is taken, you won't be able to close your eyes and they'll get dry and irritated easily. Show your surgeon younger photos of yourself to prevent this problem. To correct this, unsightly skin grafts have to be taken from behind the ears and placed patchwork in the upper eyelid area. Not good.

Lasts For

Eyelid surgery should last for many years if done properly.

Terry Tip

Pick an experienced surgeon who is thoughtful and careful, as this procedure, although technically easy, can go very wrong in inexperienced or rushed hands.

Face—Full Facelift

The big daddy of all facial cosmetic surgery. This is my favorite procedure. Done properly, it can give a wonderful, natural look that turns the clock back ten or even twenty years. Improperly done, it's a disaster and subject of much mockery and gossiping. Who hasn't tittered about some celebrity who "took a break" and came back to work with a face altered beyond recognition? Or stretched so tight you could practically bounce silver dollars off her cheeks? Or who looks preternaturally smooth and taut when she's old enough to be your grandmother?

Those are the crummy facelifts. A good one, on the other hand, can do wonders for those who have despaired of their wrinkles and sagging. You will look more relaxed, revitalized, and years younger—like yourself. You won't look decades younger and you shouldn't want to, but you'll look more *youthful*. That's as good as it gets.

What It Does

Facelifts are extremely effective for fixing sagging, droopy skin, especially in the mid-face and double chin/chin jowls; reducing creases below the lower eyelids; and addressing wrinkles around the nose, mouth, and chin, such as the nasolabial folds, smile lines, marionette lines, and smoker's lines. Fat often becomes displaced with age and may create jowls along the jawline and what appears to be a double chin. The facelift removes or repositions these fat deposits and tightens the underlying muscles so your mid-face and jawline are smooth and taut. But, hopefully, not *too* taut!

How It's Done

The natural fat (properly called the malar fat pads) you have in your face that once gave you such chubby cheeks naturally descends with age. (Yes, gravity sucks!) For the traditional full facelift, incisions are made within the hairline, beginning at the temples, and extend down and around the backs of the ears into the hairline in the lower scalp. A less invasive technique that uses shorter incisions may be used—this will depend on your facial structure and the degree of correction needed. Once the facial tissues are uplifted, the skin is re-draped over the new contours and excess skin is removed.

Realistic Expectations

Facelifts are the go-to procedure when you have loose skin and wrinkles that can't be fixed with lasers or fillers. How well a facelift will work depends on a lot of variables, and that includes the elasticity of your skin. Facelifts will almost be more successful when you have them in your forties or fifties and your skin is still fairly firm, but there is no upper end for doing one as long as you're in good health and don't smoke. My oldest facelift patient was ninety-four!

Pain Meter

4–7. It hurts, but using newer techniques focused on muscle tightening and long-acting numbing medicine, it is extremely well tolerated. Your face has been cut open and rearranged. You will be given prescription pain meds and you should take them! The level of pain should start to diminish after two to three days.

Recuperation Time

A facelift is not minor surgery. After the procedure, your face will be bandaged, and you will be closely monitored in a recovery area. Drainage tubes may be placed to remove any blood or fluid that collects under the skin. You'll need to sleep on a lot of pillows to keep your head elevated. You will need at least a week to recuperate, and most of my patients can go back to work then. You can resume strenuous activities after about four weeks.

Possible Complications/What Can Go Wrong

The facelift, although generally very safe and in reliable hands, can go very badly in a lot of different ways. Complications are divided into two general categories: early and late. Early complications include excessive bleeding, nerve damage changing the way your face moves, numbness, and pain. Late complications include permanent nerve damage, scarring, facial distortion, and a bizarre altered look if improperly done.

Lasts For

Years. I've found that women whose lifts were a bit too tight at first can sometimes look really wonderful a year or two after the surgery, when the muscles have softened a bit. Typically, a good facelift done early can last ten to fifteen years before a touch-up is needed.

Terry Tip

Do it early, when you first start forming loose and jowly skin. It will last longer and your recuperation will be easier.

Forehead Lift

The brow and forehead are some of the first areas on your face to develop lines, wrinkles, and drooping, and these effects of aging often make you look tired, sad, or even angry when you're not. Brow lift surgery, or a forehead lift, can fix that.

What It Does

A forehead lift can fix drooping brows that may cover the upper eyelids; horizontal lines across your forehead and on the bridge of your nose; and the glabellar or frown lines between your brows that you may have tried to erase with Botox.

How It's Done

With the traditional technique, an incision behind the hairline at the top of the head is used to lift the skin on the forehead and adjust the tissue and muscle underneath. A less-invasive technique uses an endoscope, which is a thin tube with a camera attached to the end. Special instruments are placed through a few short incisions in the scalp and used to adjust the tissue and muscle beneath the skin.

Realistic Expectations

Many of my patients get a forehead lift when they're already planning to be on the table for a facelift (which corrects only the mid-face and chin area) and/or eyelid surgery, so they don't have to go through the recuperation period several times.

Pain Meter

4–7. It can be surprisingly painful.

Recuperation Time

Your forehead will be bandaged and wrapped to reduce swelling and bruising. You need to keep your head elevated, and no vigorous movement, for at least a full week. Most patients are able to return to work and normal activities at that point. No strenuous exercise for at least four weeks afterward, too.

Possible Complications/What Can Go Wrong

Complications include hair loss, scalp numbing, scarring, and recurrent drooping.

Lasts For

Seven to ten years.

Terry Tip

If you look great when you manually raise your brows with your fingers, strongly consider it. Otherwise, intermittent Botox injections can make moderate improvements in brow elevation, and it's better to avoid this procedure if possible.

Nose—Rhinoplasty

The nose changes as we age. The bones in the upper part of the nose stay constant but the cartilage in the tip continues to grow. This often results in a droopy tip, and the distance between the upper lip and the nose shortens. That makes us look older.

What It Does

Rhinoplasty is surgery of the nose that can correct a range of cosmetic and/or functional issues. The shape and size of almost any characteristic of the nose can be improved, including the tip, nostrils, bridge, angle between the nose and upper lip, and the overall projection. Rhinoplasty can also correct structural defects within the nasal passage, such as a deviated septum, that impair breathing; that's a medical rather than a cosmetic procedure, and is called a septoplasty. (A lot of patients try to use the "messed-up deviated septum" scenario to see if their insurance companies will cover the procedure, but they need a genuine problem for that to work!)

How It's Done

With an open rhinoplasty technique, an inconspicuous incision is made along the thin strip of tissue between the nostrils (columella). Once the skin can be lifted, the underlying structures of the nose can be reshaped. With the closed rhinoplasty technique, incisions are hidden within the nostrils, and there are no visible scars.

Realistic Expectations

Your nose is definitely going to be different. It is far better for your nose to have a gentle reshaping than a drastic change that is extremely hard to fix, even if it doesn't seem so at first, because it can take a long time for the swelling to completely go down so you can make an accurate judgment.

Another issue is that the esthetics of a nose shape are so completely subjective. You need to have a serious talk with your surgeon before the procedure about what to expect. *Always* scrutinize his or her before/after photos. Are the noses all shaped the same? Is that what you really want, even if it might not be best for your face?

I've found that the patients who want an improved version of their own nose end up the happiest. Problems arise when patients want a nose like someone else that has no remote relationship to the way their nose looks. The best way to think about your nose is to divide it into the bridge and the tip. The key to the tip is reducing it to a reasonable size rather than trying to sculpt it; there are limitations to the changes we can make due to variables like skin thickness, tip projection, and nostril length. The key to the bridge is to not make it too narrow or too low. Leaving a little bump makes it look completely natural sometimes and prevents the "operated" look.

Pain Meter

5–7. Nose jobs where the bone inside is "broken" and the cartilage reshaped are painful for a few days, but you should respond well to pain meds.

Recuperation Time

Your nose will be covered with bandages, and packing or a splint will be placed inside your nose to support it as it heals, and removed at about five days. Most patients return to work after one week; most swelling usually takes a few weeks to resolve. You need to be on restricted activities during that time. Expect your nose to continue to change slightly over the next year as it heals and the swelling finally goes down.

Possible Complications/What Can Go Wrong

Bleeding, infection, and scarring occur but are pretty rare in rhinoplasty surgery.

The biggest complication with rhinoplasty, however, is that the job was botched. Not physically, but *esthetically*. If you have a distinctive nose, think carefully before moving forward. You might be thrilled and you might be devastated, and if you miss your old nose or need to do *something*, revision rhinoplasty might be an option. Bear in mind that revision rhinoplasty will always be much more complicated and take more time to perform because there will be scar tissue inside. Entire nasal structures may need reshaping, and the soft tissues of the nose may not respond well to additional surgery, the healing process (which can sometimes take up to two years), and the resulting inflammation. In some cases, cartilage grafts are needed to support or define the new nasal shape. These are taken from your own body, most often from the nasal septum, the ear, or near the sternum from the ribs. In other cases, synthetic materials can be used to support the new structure and shape of the nose.

Lasts For

A nose job is permanent, but along with everything else that gravity affects as decades go by, you might see your nose subtly getting a bit longer as you age.

Terry Tip

Nose jobs are great, but *under-do* it! It's far better to have a slightly underdone nose that isn't perfect than an overly narrowed sculpted one that people can't stop staring at.

Plastic Surgery Procedures—Body

Arms—Arm Lift

Bat wings. Bingo arms. Flag-flappers. I hear all kinds of nicknames for the lax skin on the upper arms, as this is an area of the body that really bothers a lot of women. The skin there often loses elasticity sooner than in other parts of the body; even working out with weights sometimes doesn't help. If so, an arm lift may be an option.

What It Does

Tightens arm skin from the armpit to the elbow.

How It's Done

There are two types, depending on where and how loose the skin is. If the lax skin is only from the armpit to halfway to the elbow, a limited-incision brachialplasty, or arm lift, can be done. This leaves a scar primarily only in the armpit. If you have laxity all the way to the elbow, then a full-length scar from armpit to elbow will result. Think carefully before electing to do the full arm lift. It's a big, long scar, and if it doesn't heal perfectly it'll probably be worse than the original loose skin. I reserve this full lift for people who have lost a ton of weight and the arm laxity is significant.

Realistic Expectations

You should have tighter skin and visible scars (full lift).

Pain Meter

2–3.

Recuperation Time

Two weeks of limited arm use.

Possible Complications/What Can Go Wrong

Scarring and more scarring. Surgery on extremities has a higher complication rate of infection, wounds splitting open, and stitches coming undone.

Lasts For

This is permanent if you keep your weight steady.

Terry Tip

As a busy plastic surgeon I probably do two a month. Most plastic surgeons, however, do one or two a *year*. Research carefully. I would express caution with this procedure. It's less than perfect.

Belly—Tummy Tuck

If you have skin on your abdomen that just won't tighten up, even with regular exercise and a healthy diet—usually due to multiple pregnancies and/or weight loss—a tummy tuck can help.

What It Does

Tummy tuck surgery, or abdominoplasty, is a procedure designed to noticeably improve the appearance of the stomach area.

How It's Done

A full tummy tuck removes excess skin and fat while tightening the abdominal wall muscles. After the remaining skin is re-draped, the navel may also be repositioned. A partial or mini tummy tuck focuses on removing just the excess skin and fat below the navel.

Realistic Expectations

Ideal candidates for a tummy tuck are in relatively good health and have permanently stretched skin and stubborn fat deposits in their abdominal area. Like liposuction, a tummy tuck is not a weight-loss procedure.

I've had a lot of patients who've undergone the time, expense, and pain of a mini tummy tuck and it didn't work—it is one of the most misused operations in plastic surgery, and only a very small percentage of patients benefit from one. This is because if you tighten the lower stomach only, the upper stomach will now bulge. Most patients are better served by a full tummy tuck with abdominal muscle tightening all the way up to the chest.

The major downside is the *scar*. Emphasis on the word *scar*, because when I see a patient for a tummy tuck consult, although I do hundreds a year, I want him or her to first be confronted with the discussion about the hip-to-hip *scar*. Although it's low and usually very fine lined, it's a very long *scar* that may develop thickening or keloids and may need revision, as the wound is under tension and that predisposes it to *scar* widening or thickening. If that doesn't scare you away, then I think it is one of the most satisfying procedures in plastic surgery, and generally patients absolutely love the outcome. However, there is a long *scar*. Hey, I want to make sure you really get that! A really long *scar*!

Pain Meter

6–8 down to 2–3. Tummy tucks are one of the most painful of all the plastic surgery procedures—it's major abdominal surgery. Since your core is responsible for all movement (and that includes breathing), every time you move, you're going to feel it. However, there is a trick your surgeon can use. He or she can place a pain pump inside the tummy-skin area that infuses a local anesthetic post-op for three to five days afterward. This cuts the pain way down; that, along with oral pain meds, makes the recovery very doable.

Recuperation Time

Most patients can return to work seven to ten days after surgery and usually make a nearly full recovery after about a month—but for some it can take up to six months to fully recover. You shouldn't do any heavy lifting (kids, laundry, etc.) at all during recovery.

Possible Complications/What Can Go Wrong

Okay, are you ready for this? Although it's an extremely common procedure with a very high satisfaction rate, it's also the *most dangerous* operation in plastic surgery. It's the one operation that puts you at a significantly higher risk of one of the most dreaded and dangerous complications, the pulmonary embolism. This is a clot that has formed in your lower venous system and broken off into the bloodstream and has now "embolized" or traveled to your lungs, where it blocks important vessels. If untreated even for a short period of time, it can be fatal—when you hear of someone dying after a plastic surgery procedure, it's almost always due to a pulmonary embolism.

Here's the good news. It's rare and occurs in only about one out of every 1,000 tummy tucks. If you and your surgeon watch closely for any signs of it, like sudden shortness of breath or anxiety, then the chances of dying are more like one in 150,000.

Lasts For

A tummy tuck should give you permanent results as long as you maintain your weight and don't have any future pregnancies.

Terry Tip

Before proceeding with a tummy tuck, look at lots of pictures online showing the *scars*, make sure your surgeon is a good belly-button maker (look at his photos), and if you feel short of breath after surgery, go straight to the ER and tell them you think you have a pulmonary embolism. Do these things and you will be fine.

Breast Lift—For Sagging

It's bad enough that gravity pulls down our faces and our butts. What about a woman's breasts? They're not immune from it either, and those whose breasts are large or are naturally shaped with a downward turn can not only be unhappy as time goes by, but suffer from discomfort and shoulder pain from bras that don't fit.

What It Does

Also known as a mastopexy, this surgery adds a more attractive contour to the breasts by eliminating sagging skin and excess tissue. Breasts sag due to pregnancy and breast-feeding, weight fluctuations, gravity, genetics, and doing a lot of bouncing or jarring exercising over the years without good support. Unlike breast augmentation, a breast lift focuses on altering the position and shape of the breasts, rather than just improving fullness and volume.

How It's Done

There are four types of breast lift:

❖ Crescent lift. This is the least invasive and good for very minor sagging and nipples that point downward. Incisions are made on the upper half of the areolas, so scarring is practically nonexistent. It's often combined with breast augmentation.

❖ Benelli or circumareolar lift. This procedure is best when there is slight sagging and asymmetry in the nipples. Incisions are around the areolas, so there should be no noticeable scars. It should only be used with breast implants, as it tends to flatten the breast mound.

❖ Lollipop lift. Used for moderate sagging and the nipples pointing downward, this lift allows for tightening the breast tissue and repositioning the nipples and areolas. There will be small scarring.

❖ Anchor lift. The most invasive procedure, used for significant sagging and downward-pointing nipples. This is so more breast tissue and skin can be removed, the breast tissue can be tightened, and the areolas and nipples repositioned. This procedure leaves scars around the areola, down the front part of the breast vertically, and in the horizontal crease where the breast meets the stomach.

Realistic Expectations

The big questions in breast lift surgery are always what lift do you need and is there any way to do a smaller lift with less scarring and still get good results? It works like this:

1. If your nipple is at or slightly below the breast crease, then a small implant with no lift is the best option.

2. If the nipple is an inch or more below the breast/chest crease, then you need a lift plus or minus implants.

3. If you don't want to be any bigger, then a lift alone can work.

4. If you have decent volume in the middle third of your breast, then a vertical or full lift will work great.

5. If you have no volume in the upper or middle of your breasts, then the best option is often an implant with a lift. Never allow a Benelli lift without an implant.

Many of my patients choose to have a breast lift and augmentation at the same time, so they can have firm breasts in the size of their choosing. This combination does increase your risk of the nipple dying due to poor blood supply, and you may have seen me on *Botched* using leeches in this situation. Bear in mind that a simultaneous breast augmentation and implants is a very *advanced*, tricky operation. You need a good surgeon. A high percentage of our *Botched* applicants have bad problems related to having these two procedures together.

Pain Meter

1–2. Breast lifts are surprisingly painless.

Recuperation Time

If not using implants with the lift, it has a very fast recovery of three to five days on average.

Possible Complications/What Can Go Wrong

Scarring and nipple loss are the two big ones. It's not uncommon to need a scar revision after a lift because parts of the wound healed with more noticeable scars. I think it wise to go into a breast lift prepared for the possibility of a small scar revision six to nine months later.

Lasts For

Breast lifts should last for years as long as you have no future pregnancies or large weight fluctuations, or put in large, heavy breast implants.

Terry Tip

Try at all costs to avoid a lift. You can always put scars on your breast later with a more formal lift if needed, but once they are there, they are there forever.

Breast Augmentation—For Size and Shape

The size and shape of your breasts are determined by genetics. Sure, if you gain a lot of weight your breast size will increase along with the rest of you, but other than that, you have no control over how your breasts look and feel, and there's no special diet or exercise that can significantly increase the volume of your breasts. This leaves a lot of women very unhappy with their breasts, especially if they are small, asymmetrical (which is very common), a different shape or volume after pregnancy and breast-feeding, or seemingly out of proportion to their figures. Enter the augmentation. It is definitely an anti-aging procedure, as it makes your breasts look as firm and shapely as they may have been when you were much younger (lots of my patients call them "perky!"), and I would choose this over the breast lift when age has done a number on your breasts because the scars are barely a factor in comparison to how bad they can be with a lift.

What It Does

Breast augmentation surgery places implants inside the breasts to improve their size and shape. It can help minor degrees of sagging but anything more will require a breast lift, which is why I often do both procedures at once.

How It's Done

There are four key variables to consider for breast augmentation: incision location, pocket location, type of implant, and size.

The best incision procedures are to place them around the lower outline of the areola, along the crease on the underside of the breast, within the natural fold of armpit, or within the navel, where the implant is tunneled up to the breast. The pocket used to place the implants comes in subglandular (below the breast, on top of the muscle) or submuscular (below the pectoralis major muscle—usually the best placement). Although the recovery is longer, submuscular implants have a lower complication rate and look better. This placement also means you should still be able to breast-feed, too.

There are several kinds of implants:

❖ Saline implants. These consist of an outer silicone shell filled with a saltwater solution. They're FDA-approved for breast augmentation in women eighteen years and older. Saline implants feel slightly firmer than natural breast tissue and present no health risk if a rupture occurs. Very few patients in my practice choose saline anymore. Although they were once considered the "safe" implant, they actually have a higher complication rate than a silicone implant, and the cosmetic result isn't as good as with silicone.

❖ Silicone implants. FDA-approved for breast augmentation in women over the age of twenty-three (the FDA can be very arbitrary with ages!), these implants are made of 100 percent pure-grade silicone gel. They tend to look and feel more like natural breast tissue than saline implants and are less likely to rupture. In my opinion, silicone implants are far and away better than saline both in terms of cosmetic result and complications.

❖ Shaped implants. Implants now come in different shapes according to how filled they are and how much they project. The hot thing now is higher profile implants that are "extra full." These implants have the lowest chance of being able to feel them in people with thin skin and little breast tissue. They also aren't as wide and tend to give less of a "side boob" look.

You need to discuss the pros and cons of implants with your surgeon. Silicone implants were pulled off the market by the FDA in 1992 due to safety fears, and after extensive studies were reapproved in 2006. But silicone is still a foreign substance, and anyone with a silicone implant is instructed to have an MRI every other year to assess whether or not it's ruptured. (An MRI is very expensive and rarely covered by insurance, but it's the only way to assess whether a silicone implant is still intact or not.) Don't forget: the size you choose is absolutely critical, too!

Realistic Expectations

You'll see the results right after your surgery, but the implants may sit high on your chest for the first few months until they settle into a more natural position. With new techniques, we can allow them to sit properly right away. In addition, postsurgical swelling may initially cause your breasts to appear larger than their final result. But they will certainly be larger and firmer.

Because breast surgery can have complications (see below); because you might not be thrilled with the size, shape, and placement of your new breasts; because you might not like how your new breasts *feel*; and because augmentation is often botched, breast revision surgery can improve the shape, size, projection, and symmetry of your breasts. Yes, it means you have to go under the knife again, but revision surgery is sometimes best when the implants need to be removed or replaced.

Pain Meter

5–7.

Recuperation Time

Approximately seven to ten days of downtime are needed after surgery with breast implants, after which you can return to work and resume normal activities. You need a lot of rest, and you need to take your pain meds. Expect a full recovery in about six weeks, and avoid any strenuous exercise, lifting, or physical activities during that time.

Possible Complications/What Can Go Wrong

I keep busy on *Botched* dealing with many different augmentation complications:

❖ Capsular contracture. This occurs when the fibrous tissue capsule that forms around the implant after surgery tightens and squeezes the implant. This is because your immune system can decide it doesn't like the implants 19 to 20 percent of the time, and it makes thick scar tissue called encapsulation around the implant, which can distort the breast, make it hard, and cause pain.

❖ Rupture. A rupture occurs when the silicone shell of an implant breaks open or tears. This warrants immediate attention, as the silicone reaction can cause significant scarring around the implant and can result in painful contracture of the surrounding tissues. With a saline implant you won't need an MRI, as there will be an obvious deflation and wrinkling in the breast. If this happens, at least you don't have to worry about the saline solution, since it's sterile and absorbed by your body.

❖ Shifting. Breasts can shift from their original position and become obviously fake and asymmetrical. While it's almost impossible to achieve perfect breast symmetry, poor breast shape is usually due to poor surgical technique.

❖ Rippling. If your breasts are very small and/or you don't have enough natural breast tissue to cover the implant, or if the implant chosen is too large, there can be visible implant rippling or wrinkling through the skin.

If you're unhappy or had complications, your original surgeon might not be the best person to perform your revision surgery if he or she is not highly experienced in implant removal. Find a specialist in breast revision, as this surgeon is more likely to achieve optimum results with reduced risks. In most cases, patients can change to a different implant size or type as long as it does not pose a significant risk.

Lasts For

Breast implants are not considered lifetime devices and will likely need to be replaced at some point. It's impossible to tell when, as individual circumstances will determine this.

Terry Tip

As for the OMG Fake Factor, the best augmentation is one that doesn't look artificial, like two "bolt-ons." The best result, in my opinion, is a mid to full C cup and using silicone, as the feel of the implants is more like that of a regular breast. If your natural amount of breast tissue is small and your skin is tight, then sometimes it's even best to stay in the B range to prevent that high, tight look and to minimize chances of complications. The human body is not stupid and if you put a large implant in a tight, small space, it will rebel and fight back with painful scar tissue. Choose a reasonable, non-greedy-size silicone implant inserted through an incision under your areola and placed under the muscle.

Buttocks—Implants

Are your butt cheeks starting to droop the way your face cheeks are? Is your butt driving you crazy even if you work out all the time? You already learned about the fat transfer, aka the Brazilian butt lift, on page 89 in chapter 5. If you don't want the fat transfer, the other option is to get implants. But it's not an option I usually approve, as buttock implants have a very significant risk for going to crap (pun intended!).

What It Does

Usually a buttock implant is inserted through a small, two-inch incision in the cleft or "crack" between the butt cheeks. Surgeons adept at this operation will choose the intramuscular (inside the muscle) technique. Untrained surgeons place them on top of the muscle because it's an easier operation, but this usually leads to a high risk of scar tissue formation called encapsulation and can cause the implants to shift position.

How It's Done

A buttock implant is designed to increase the projection of the upper half of the buttock and give a more "bubble" butt appearance. It's best for a person with a flat buttock.

Realistic Expectations

Although we are all familiar with the skinny celebrities who have gone from no butt to huge junk-in-the-trunk overnight, butt implants are best suited for those who want a moderate improvement in projection in order to minimize the risks from placing a very large implant.

Pain Meter

7–9. Oddly it's actually a significantly painful operation, and usually lots of narcotics are needed for about a week.

Recuperation Time

This operation requires a significant recovery period. You can't sit on the area for at least a week and every little movement is agony for about two weeks. It's truly a pain in the butt.

Possible Complications/What Can Go Wrong

On *Botched* we are seeing so many complications from buttock implants that we labeled season three "the Year of the Butt." Every imaginable thing that can go wrong often does. We had a woman in season one who could completely flip hers over 360 degrees, leading to severe pain and an unacceptable appearance. The main problem is that although the implants may at first be acceptable, they can migrate, get infected, cause fluid to form around them, create a buildup of scar tissue, and cause numbness and pain.

Lasts For

If done modestly and expertly, the implants should last a lifetime once healed.

Terry Tip

If you decide to have buttock augmentation, use your own fat if you have enough in your thighs and stomach. It's a much more reliable procedure and has fewer complications. If you have low body fat, consider doing a lot of squats to build up your gluteal muscles. If that doesn't work, go to a very experienced surgeon and ask for a moderate-sized implant placed inside the muscle.

Heather: Even though I'm married to a plastic surgeon, I've always looked for nonsurgical solutions to anti-aging. I know, I know, some of you won't believe this—but if you Google me you'll find photos of me from birth until now to prove my point. Still, I'm clearly not opposed to plastic surgery when done by a board-certified plastic surgeon on an appropriate candidate with realistic expectations. As Terry says, "It's a scalpel, not a magic wand." I'm amazed at the work my husband does, and I have many friends who are the happiest they've ever been after going under the knife. Never say never—someday I may want a little nip and tuck, but until then I think I'm doing just fine. It's all about expectations and balance. Let *Botched* be your cautionary tale to do your due diligence and attain the best results possible.

PART

III

Dr. and Mrs. Guinea Pig Ratings

CHAPTER
8

Rating the Best Anti-Aging Skincare, Treatments, and Procedures

This chapter lists the best skincare and procedures for all your skincare and aging concerns, listed from least invasive to most invasive, and categorized as follows:

❖ OTC products and esthetician treatments

❖ Prescription-only products

❖ MD treatments and procedures (should only be done by board-certified dermatologists and/or plastic surgeons)

❖ Plastic surgery procedures (done only by board-certified plastic surgeons)

How to Use Our Ratings

Don't panic when you start to see visible changes in your skin! Start slow, trying OTC products or minimally invasive procedures, and avoid harsh treatments that can inadvertently age and damage your skin far more than if you'd been gentler. Always look for the nonsurgical anti-aging solutions *first*, but realize that sometimes the surgical solution *is* the solution!

The ratings in this chapter go from one to four guinea pigs. We both rated the OTC products and Terry rated the rest. They are not about which of the skincare products listed works best. Instead, they will show you how all the products and treatments stack up *against each other* for your skincare issue.

For example, for facial wrinkles, a silk pillowcase (🐹 🐹) is nearly as effective as a wrinkle cream (🐹 🐹 🐹), but not as effective as Botox (🐹 🐹 🐹 🐹) or fillers (🐹 🐹 🐹 🐹). An under-eye cream to remove puffiness might help (🐹 🐹), but a blepharoplasty (🐹 🐹 🐹 🐹) will *always* remove the bags.

We have not listed pricing, even though this is an important component. For one thing, prices constantly change for skincare products, and there is such a large price range. (Moisturizers can cost from $5 to $1,000!) Ditto for treatments. In addition, medical professionals in smaller cities with smaller overheads charge less than those in larger cities in states with high malpractice insurance rates. Surgeons with less experience might charge less than famous practitioners but be no less skilled. That's why it's so important to be a savvy consumer and comparison shop. The money and skin you save will definitely be your own!

Skincare for Your Face

Since I'm married to a plastic surgeon and I'm a television personality, I have access to basically every line of skincare on the planet. Sometimes samples come in so fast that it becomes like that pile of magazines I can never seem to get to, so I end up giving them away to our babysitter or friends. A good product can make someone feel like an absolute princess, especially if she doesn't usually have access to these items or doesn't want to splurge on herself. I love when my friends start using superior products—they realize what they've been missing.

Does this mean the product has to cost a lot or be a famous brand? Of course not. Don't buy into the latest celebrity touting some gazillion-dollar cream that's made from the eye of a newt or piglet placenta. Instead, use this chapter as if I were in your living room and we were having a girls' night *in*, where, if you're like my squad, it becomes a discussion of what to do to feel and stay young and gorgeous, and what everyone is using now.

A few general tips:

1. Focus on what you really need. Do you need luxurious packaging or to spend a lot? If the placebo effect makes you think it's worth it and you can afford it, then buy what you like! Just remember that every person has unique skincare needs; what works on your sister might not do anything for you! Identify your concerns and only buy targeted products.

2. Don't get stuck in a skincare rut. Not only does the skincare industry constantly evolve and launch effective new products, but your skin is always evolving, too. Your skincare needs at forty or fifty will be very different from what they were when you were younger.

3. Only try one product at a time, and give it a chance to work. One of my best friends is a self-proclaimed "product whore" and she literally goes from product to product, and there's no way she can tell what really works. If her skin reacts, how will she know what caused it? In my enthusiasm to start feeding my twins baby food when they were six months old, I went too fast and my son got a rash. I had to go back to bland rice cereal and start over, introducing one food at a time, waiting a week or two to see if there were any reactions, and then moving on to the next. Ugh—what a pain!

   Do the same thing with your skin—hit the reset button, especially if you've gotten irritated or had breakouts from a new product in the past. During your reset, try using Cetaphil as a cleanser and Eucerin cream as a moisturizer. They are super-gentle, fragrance-free, and dermatologist-recommended for the most sensitive skin. Once your skin is back to normal, you can keep using them or try something else.

   Some of our Consult Beaute products offer immediate results, some have a cumulative effect, and some take a few weeks for desired results. As a general rule, you should start seeing results in three to four weeks. (Yes, that is a whole month!) Be patient. If after a month you're still not seeing a significant difference, that product is likely not working for you.

4. When trying a skincare line, you don't have to buy everything at once. Choose one product to see if you like the quality, the scent, the texture, and, most of all, its effectiveness. If it works, then chances are pretty good that the rest of the line will be well tolerated by your skin. I look for the words "proprietary ingredients." That means it's formulated specifically for that product and you can't get it in those strengths or combinations anywhere else. Purchase that product first.

   Chapter 3 taught you how to *read the label*, so do it!

5. Know who you're buying from. It is about who you trust! A solid company with many years of producing quality products or a plastic surgeon, dermatologist, or esthetician creating products makes sense. An infomercial, flyer, or ad in a magazine with nothing to back up sensationalized claims is probably not worth your time.

6. Yes, you can return your product! I know—you're scared, embarrassed, the salesperson at the counter spent a lot of time helping you . . . whatever the reason, get over it. Companies want to know if their products are effective or if you have a negative reaction. Even if you used up most of the product, it is still returnable. Realize, though, that where you shop is important because it can make a difference with the returns policy. Choose wisely. If you're buying online, be sure to check the small print so you don't get stuck with shipping fees that cost more than the product!

7. Ask for samples. Don't be shy. A regular sample size will only give you enough product for a day or two, so you can't accurately judge its true efficacy. What you can tell is if you like the smell and texture, which are very important since our touch and olfactory senses are crucial to our overall skincare experience.

I'll say it again: *don't fall for the hype!* Ads are Photoshopped and claims can be bogus. Trust your judgment. There is no magic skincare bullet—are there diamonds from Tiffany hidden inside?—but there sure are a lot of magical claims!

Anti-Aging: Acne Care

OTC Acne Products

Hype or Hot

As you learned on pages 60–61 in chapter 4, Terry's combination of glycolic acid, salicylic acid, and benzoyl peroxide effectively treats acne—and what will heat up treatment is *cold*. Ice is the best and the cheapest OTC anti-inflammatory ever! Using ice to cool down your face before applying the benzoyl peroxide, and applying a cold pack afterward, is the crucial step.

Recommended Brands

Salicylic Acid Cleanser: Clean and Clear Advantage Acne Control 3-in-1 Foaming Wash, Clearogen Foaming Cleanser, Murad Acne Complex Clarifying Cleanser, Neutrogena Oil-Free Acne Wash Cream Cleanser, Yes to Tomatoes Detoxifying Charcoal Cleanser

Glycolic Acid Lotion: Alpha Hydrox Enhanced Lotion 10% Glycolic, Aqua Glycolic Face Cream, Malin + Goetz Resurfacing 10% Glycolic Acid Pads, MD Forté Glycolic Acid Facial Lotion III, Peter Thomas Roth AHA/BHA Acne Clearing Gel

Benzoyl Peroxide: Acne.org 8 oz. Treatment, Claror Acne Treatment, Jan Marini Acne Treatment Wash, Neutrogena On-the-Spot Acne Treatment, Paula's Choice Clear Regular Strength Daily Skin Clearing Treatment

Rating: 🐹 🐹 🐹 🐹

Prescription Topicals

Hype or Hot

Most prescription products for acne are retinoid-based, the best-known being Retin-A (or tretinoin), Differin, and Tazorac.

FDA-approved for acne, they also have a potent anti-aging effect (see pages 106–107). Each has advantages and disadvantages best reviewed with your dermatologist.

Rating: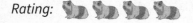

Prescription Antibiotics and/or Accutane

Hype or Hot

Antibiotics such as tetracycline, clindamycin, erythromycin, and doxycycline are sometimes used for acne, so discuss with your dermatologist, as there can be side effects from long-term use. Accutane is a retinoid that's usually more effective, especially for intractable, cystic acne, and the only way to potentially cure acne, as it completely changes the production of oil from the sebaceous glands; with no oil plugging, acne cannot occur. It also has the most serious potential side effects like liver failure and is extremely toxic to developing fetuses, so it must never be used if you are considering a pregnancy or actually pregnant.

Heather: When I was twenty-seven, I suddenly got acne. I tried OTC products to no avail, so my dermatologist put me on Accutane. It worked, but I was put on a short-term high dose, which I didn't know was counterproductive over the long run because my acne returned several years later. This time, I went on a lower dose for much longer. I was skeptical, but my skin blossomed once the zits went away. It looked incredible—a total reboot!

Rating: for Accutane

Lasers

Hype or Hot

For acne, lasers are designed to damage the *P. acnes* bacteria. Acne laser centers are everywhere, expensive, and can be effective for treating certain types of inflammatory acne, but are relatively ineffective against the usual variety of blackheads and zits. Much better to buy a generic bottle of benzoyl peroxide that will kill more bacteria better than any $100,000 acne laser!

Rating:

Light Therapy

Hype or Hot

In-office and at-home light therapy is a big business, using blue or red light to destroy acne bacteria much like lasers are designed to do. Certain light spectrums have also been touted as reducing oil production, which is the holy grail of acne treatments like Accutane. Do they work? In four words: kinda sorta not really. It's the same as the laser above, plus they require at least ten to twenty short treatments. They basically are what we call in the medical profession a "wallet biopsy." Pass.

Rating:

Peels

Hype or Hot

Peels containing alpha hydroxy acids like salicylic or glycolic acid can be a very important part of an acne regimen, working wonders on acne-prone skin and as a preventative measure to keep acne away. I recommend at least a glycolic acid peel of 30 (light) to 50 (medium) percent and a 30 percent salicylic acid strength, at least every two to four weeks.

Rating:

Anti-Aging: Dry Skin

Moisturizers, Oils, and Serums

Hype or Hot

Look, I like luxe as much as anyone, but after trying just about every moisturizer in the world, I'm happy to report that there are drugstore brands that are just as or even *more* effective as the costly brands, especially if they contain the same ingredients. Spend your money on treatment creams, and use a moisturizer that gets the job done without breaking the bank.

Recommended Brands

Creams for Face: Aveeno Clear Complexion Daily Moisturizer, Belif—The True Cream Moisturizing Bomb, Biologique Recherche Crème Hydravit'S, Bliss Drench 'n' Quench, Consult Beaute Volumagen Concentrate and Cream, Dr. Hauschka Revitalizing Day Cream, Erno Laszlo Phormula 3-9 Repair Cream and/or White Marble Translucence Cream, Neutrogena Hydro Boost Water Gel

Oils: Bobbi Brown Extra Face Oil, Ole Henriksen Pure Truth Vitamin C Youth Activating Oil, Kahina Giving Beauty Argan Oil, Meaningful Beauty Vitality Oil, Sunday Riley Artemis Hydroactive Cellular Face Oil

Creams for Body: Ahava Mineral Body Lotion, Bliss Body Butter Maximum Moisture Cream, L'Occitane Ultra Rich Body Cream in Shea Butter, Suave Sea Mineral Infusion Hand and Body Lotion, Tatcha Indigo Soothing Silk Body Butter

Masks: Ahava Hydration Cream Mask, AmorePacific Moisture Bound Sleeping Recovery Mask, Boscia Tsubaki Deep Hydration Sleeping Mask, Consult Beaute Volumagen Re-Imaging Beaute Treatment, Korres Advanced Brightening Sleeping Facial

Rating:

Anti-Aging: Loss of Firmness and Elasticity, Sagging, and Crepey Skin on Your Face

Firming Products

Hype or Hot

Some brands can do wonders if you need a lift for a few hours. Don't expect long-term results because once your skin's elasticity starts to go, no topical product can reverse this.

Recommended Brands

Lifting Creams: By Terry Liftessence Rich Cream, Caudalíe Resveratrol Lift Night Infusion Cream, Cellex-C Advanced-C Skin Tightening Cream, Kanebo Sensai Cellular Performance Lifting Radiance Cream, Olay Regenerist Micro-Sculpting Cream Moisturizer, Perricone MD Re:Firm, Age Perfect Cell Renewal Cream, Philosophy Ultimate Miracle Worker, Vichy Liftactiv Supreme

Instant, Temporary Lift: Charlotte's Magic Cream, DermaSilk 5 Minute Face Lift and/or Flawless Erase, Ren Flash Rinse 1 Minute Facial, Revitalift Volume Filler, Roloxin Lift, StriVectin High-Potency Wrinkle Filler

Rating: 🐹 🐹 🐹

Botox

Hype or Hot

Botox is the granddaddy of wrinkle removers, primarily from the nose up to the forehead. But as wonderful as it can be, it can also give you a shiny, overly plastic appearance. This is particularly true with foreheads that are very high or very round. It's not only weird looking, it's also like wearing a Botox ad on your face. I really hate that look!

Rating: 🐹 🐹 🐹 🐹 *for wrinkle removal,* 🐹 *if overused*

Fillers

Hype or Hot

Just as Botox is used for lines above the nose, fillers are generally used for lines below the nose, most commonly the deep lines from the nose to the lips (nasolabial folds) and the corner of the lips to the chin (marionette lines). The most popular fillers, Juvéderm and Restylane, made from hyaluronic acid, last around five months. (Doctors will tell you more—not true!) If done before the skin is too saggy they work really well. Best is a max of 1 cc syringe in the upper and 1 cc in the lower. Radiesse is useful for the mid-face and cheeks and can last as long as a year. Sculptra requires three or more treatments and is designed to induce your own body to form collagen (I love this one) in the temple and cheek area. Voluma is incredibly useful for the hollows in the cheek area. Be sure to read the section on pages 92–97 in chapter 5— fillers can have serious complications!

Rating: 🐹 🐹 🐹 🐹

Light Therapy

Hype or Hot

Although hyped for skin tightening, don't bother using IPL machines for anything other than improving skin tone or color, no matter what the doctor or laser nurse tells you! They are weak for sagging, at best.

Rating: 🐹

Lasers

Hype or Hot

Lasers are both extremely useful and effective in anti-aging, *and* extremely overused and ineffective depending on what you're trying to accomplish. Where they don't really work well is in the area of facial skin tightening—the classic overpromise and under-deliver scenario that laser treatments are often known for. If and *only* if the skin is in the early stages of droopiness, a fractionated CO2 laser can significantly tighten the skin and delay a facelift or need for fillers. Otherwise, lasers are not the miracle treatments for anti-aging as yet, and this is coming from a guy who in his career has purchased more than a million dollars worth of lasers! As you know, the number one reason for plastic surgery malpractice suits is due to scarring and pigmentation complications from laser treatments. Lasers are pretty good for wrinkle removal, pigment improvement, and tattoo and hair removal, but beyond that are more hype than hot.

Rating: 🐹 🐹 🐹 *only for tightening as noted*

Anti-Aging: Loss of Firmness and Elasticity, Sagging, and Crepey Skin on Your Neck

Neck Products

Hype or Hot

Unless you want to wear a turtleneck for the rest of your life, don't ignore your neck. You need a targeted product.

Recommended Brands

Algenist Firming and Lifting Neck Cream, Consult Beaute Volumagen Volumizing Neck Treatment Cream, Dr. Denese Firmatone Rx Retinol Maximum Chin and Neck Firming Serum, Isomers Neck and Chin Firming, Perricone MD Cosmeceuticals Firming Neck Therapy, Revision Nectifirm, StriVectin Tightening Neck Serum Roller. *Note:* You can also use instant firming products on page 175 here, too.

Rating: 🐹 🐹

Botox

Hype or Hot

If you have bands of muscle that get worse with animation, regular injections of Botox into those bands can dramatically tighten the neck and hold off the need for a facelift. The effects are rather amazing if the skin isn't too loose yet.

Rating: 🐹🐹🐹

Fillers

Hype or Hot

Fillers are not appropriate for use in the neck—ever!

Rating: 🚫

Radiofrequency and Ultrasound

Hype or Hot

Ultherapy is a noninvasive ultrasound that purposely causes an injury to the deeper layers of the skin, inducing the skin to use its own natural healing processes to cause tightening. While hyped as no recovery/ no downtime, in truth it's a very painful treatment that at best tightens the skin 20 to 40 percent and at worst doesn't work at all. Thermage uses noninvasive radiofrequency energy to tighten the skin and has been around much longer, but it has about the same results. Although these two methods probably represent the future of skin tightening, they are at this time expensive and only mildly effective. With low expectations, though, they can improve loose neck skin without surgery.

Rating: 🐹🐹

Lasers

Hype or Hot

Lasers are *not* to be used, as neck skin is very thin and prone to scarring and pigmentation problems.

Rating: 🚫

Anti-Aging: Wrinkles on Your Face

Anti-Wrinkle Products

Hype or Hot

Collagen and elastin are often hyped as effective ingredients in OTC products, but it's a bogus claim because collagen and elastin molecules are too big to get past the top two layers of your skin—it's absolutely impossible. No OTC product can *add* collagen or elastin to your skin.

We created a proprietary ingredient, Volumagen, made from marine collagen filling spheres and hyaluronic acid, for Consult Beaute. It works quickly and also has a cumulative effect. I like the idea of filling the skin in a natural way and using your own body's moisture to plump up your skin rather than getting fillers. Anything you can do to add volume in your face without needles is a good thing!

Recommended Brands

Consult Beaute Volumagen Facial Cream and Concentrate, Lancôme Visionnaire Advanced Skin Corrector, Neutrogena Rapid Wrinkle Repair, La Prairie Cellular Power Charge Night, RoC Multi Correxion Lift Anti-Gravity Day Moisturizer, RoC Retinol Correxion Max Wrinkle Resurfacing System, Skinceuticals Triple Lipid Restore 2:4:2

Rating: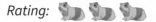

Silk Pillowcases

Hype or Hot

Hot! They're affordable luxuries and I never sleep without one. They're also great at keeping your hair silky smooth, as silk doesn't cause the same amount of static as cotton does.

Recommended Brands

Lily Silk, Slip

Rating:

Prescription Topicals

Hype or Hot

The holy grail of prescription topicals, and the only products FDA-approved for wrinkle reduction and anti-aging, are the vitamin A–based products, the oldest and best studied being Retin-A. These isotretinoins increase cell turnover, decrease collagen breakdown, help skin cells repair themselves, and even out blotchy skin. Their only problem is they also cause a significant amount of inflammation and are almost always very irritating. Newer formulations are "encapsulated" in order to minimize inflammation, but at higher doses can still cause significant redness and peeling. I recommend OTC formulations with the precursors to isotretinoins called retinols. The newer formulations, like Consult Beaute's Regenerol (3 percent retinol, the highest concentration available), are encapsulated and in a higher strength have similar effects to prescription products without the cost or side effects.

Rating: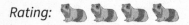

Botox

Hype or Hot

Botox is incredibly effective for wrinkles on the forehead and between the brows—the animation lines, meaning when you make expressions. It can also reduce lines at rest if the lines aren't too deep. Generally, twenty units are injected.

Rating:

Fat Transfer

Hype or Hot

Fat transfer is useful for a more permanent solution but only in very specific areas of the face, specifically the nasolabial folds and to increase the width of the cheeks as they deflate with age. Beware, however, because too much fat injected for this purpose gives a very unnatural look that celebrities were carrying around five years ago when the procedure first became popular.

Rating: 🐹 🐹 🐹

Fillers

Hype or Hot

Fillers are probably the most common and useful ways to reduce lines in the lower half of the face. Despite what doctors and the respective drug companies will tell you, Restylane and Juvéderm are equally effective and both last for five to seven months at most. Others like Radiesse or Sculptra last longer and are correspondingly more costly.

My favorite filler to restore youthful volume is Sculptra, as it induces the face to form collagen, but it requires at least three treatments separated by at least six weeks, and is very expensive. It lasts three to five years, however, and I prefer it over fat injections, which can be unpredictable and rapidly reabsorbed. Fillers do not tighten the skin, so ignore any overhyped claims for a nonsurgical "filler facelift"— see page 231 in chapter 9.

Rating: 🐹 🐹 🐹 🐹

Lasers

Hype or Hot

The fractionated CO2 laser is probably the most effective way to reduce fine lines around the eyes and mouth permanently, with less risk of scarring and pigmentation changes more common with the older CO2 lasers. They can reduce deep wrinkles by as much as 60 to 75 percent and fine lines by up to 80 percent. Keep in mind that although this treatment might be called noninvasive, the recovery (red, crusty skin that looks horrendous) can be pretty invasive!

Rating: 🐹 🐹 🐹 🐹 *for fine lines and wrinkles*

Light Therapy

Hype or Hot

IPLs work very minimally for wrinkle removal. Ignore any hype!

Rating:

Peels

Hype or Hot

High concentrations of trichloroacetic acid (TCA) and glycolic acid in peels can effectively remove fine lines and wrinkles, and used to be the go-to procedure. The problem has always been lack of control because once you place the acids on the skin, the only feedback you get is from the frosting appearance before you neutralize the acid with water. Lasers are far more precise and just as effective, so peels have all but been relegated to low-strength procedures done by aestheticians for skin freshening.

Rating:

Anti-Aging: Wrinkles Around Your Eyes

Anti-Wrinkle Eye Products

Hype or Hot

Not hype at all. The skin around your eyes is highly sensitive and tender and so, of course, are your eyes, so you need an eye product that won't irritate them. Shelling out for one ought to make you more inclined to use it, too!

Recommended Brands—Wrinkles

AmorePacific Time Response Eye Renewal Crème, Cellex-C Eye Contour Gel, ColoreScience Sunforgettable Loose Mineral Eyescreen SPF 30, Consult Beaute Regenerol Concentrate and Cream, Nuxe Eye

Cream Prodigieux, Olay Total Effects Anti-Aging Eye Treatment, SK-II Essential Power Eye Cream

Recommended Brands—Puffiness and/or Dark Circles
Consult Beaute Volumagen Eye Cream, Garnier Skin Renew Anti-Dark-Circle Roller, Korres Antiwrinkle and Antiaging Eye Cream, Lancôme Génifique Eye Light-Pearl Eye-Illuminator Youth Activating Concentrate, L'Oréal Revitalift Volume Filler and/or Triple Power Eye Treatment, Simple Kind to Eyes Soothing Eye Balm

Rating: 🐹 🐹 🐹

Botox

Hype or Hot
Botox is extremely effective at minimizing crow's feet.

Rating: 🐹 🐹 🐹 🐹

Cellulite

See the entry on page 199.

Cleansers, Toners, and Makeup Removers

Cleansers

Hype or Hot
I love our Consult Beaute cleanser because it contains vitamin C for its antioxidant properties and skin brightening as well as super-gentle exfoliating agents. A lot of my friends swear by cleansing oils, which are great for dry skin.

Recommended Brands—Regular
Cetaphil Daily Face Wash, Consult Beaute Caviar Cleanser, Hada Labo Tokyo Hydrating Facial Cleanser, Paula's Choice Resist Optimal Results Hydrating Cleanser, Peter Thomas Roth Gentle Foaming Cleanser, Sonia Kashuk Resurface Gentle Exfoliating Wash

Recommended Brands—Oils

Acure Organics Facial Cleanser Argan Oil, Avalon Organics Wrinkle Therapy Cleansing Oil, Tata Harper Nourishing Oil Cleanser, Murad Renewing Cleansing Oil, Neutrogena Ultra Light Cleansing Oil, Shiseido Ultimate Cleansing Oil, Shu Uemura Anti/Oxi Skin-Refining Cleansing Oil

Rating: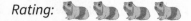

Toners

Hype or Hot

Korean skincare is super hot right now, and some of the brands make great toners, especially in spray bottles so you can spritz yourself whenever you want a sweet-smelling skin refresher.

Recommended Brands

Caudalíe Moisturizing Toner, Lancôme Tonique Confort Comforting Rehydrating Toner, Ling New York Dual Moisture Emulsion, May Coop Raw Sauce, Murad Hydro-Dynamic Quenching Essence, Whamisa Olive Leaf Mist

Rating: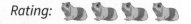

Makeup Removers

Hype or Hot

Choose one that doesn't irritate your eyes or needs a lot of scrubbing to get the mascara off. The less pulling the better. Some of the biggest brands make my eyes sting; I prefer Chanel, as it also removes my fake eyelash glue.

Recommended Brands

Caudalíe Makeup Removing Cleansing Oil, Chanel Precision Gentle Biphase Eye Makeup Remover, Clarins Instant Eye Make-Up Remover, Lancôme Bi-Facil Double-Action Eye Makeup Remover

Rating: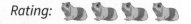

Discoloration and Hyperpigmentation

Lighteners and Brighteners

Hype or Hot

As you learned in chapter 3, I believe the worries about hydroquinone are overblown. Or, choose an active ingredient like kojic acid, azelaic acid, or vitamin C.

Recommended Brands **with Hydroquinone**

Elizabeth Arden Skin Illuminating Capsules/Emulsion/Serum, Genuine Black and White Bleaching Cream with Hydroquinone, Obagi Nu-Derm Clear Fx Skin Brightening Cream, Paula's Choice Resist Triple-Action Dark Spot Eraser, Philosophy Microdelivery Triple-Acid Brightening Peel, Porcelain Skin Whitening Serum, SkinBeauty Hydroquinone Pro Treatment

Recommended Brands **without Hydroquinone**

DDF Discoloration Reversal Moisturizer, Korres Wild Rose Advanced Brightening Sleeping Facial, Civant Skin Care Meladerm, Peter Thomas Roth Potent Botanical Skin Brightening Gel Complex, Shiseido White Lucent Brightening Moisturizing Cream

Rating: 🐹 🐹

Lasers

Hype or Hot

Lasers can be very effective for reducing pigmentation. Various lasers of differing wavelengths are used depending on your individual skin type. Most lasers are targeting the melanin-producing cells in the skin. Common lasers for the purpose are called pulsed dye lasers or YAG lasers. They can be very effective but can cause severe burning and scarring if not done by experienced laser operators who understand which skin types are at greatest risk of a complication. In general, the lighter your underlying skin color the greater chance of a successful result with the lowest chance of a complication.

Rating: 🐹 🐹 🐹 🐹

Light Therapy

Hype or Hot

Intense pulsed light or IPL, usually called a photofacial, is very effective for both improving overall skin tone, reducing pigmentation problems (such as red discoloration), and adding a youthful glow. ("Tone" is a word we use to indicate an overall evening-out of the skin color.) The darker the pigment the less effective IPL works; you generally need a laser instead.

Rating: 🐹 🐹 🐹

Peels

Hype or Hot

Jessner's solution, kojic acid, and phenol peels can be quite effective for reducing hyperpigmented areas, but have largely been replaced by lasers and IPLs.

Rating: 🐹 🐹

Dull, Blah, Sluggish Skin

Exfoliants

Hype or Hot

Your skin cell turnover slows down with age, as you know, and if you don't slough off those cells, your skin is going to look dull and blah. Try an exfoliant with gentle AHAs, or alpha hydroxy acids, as they work. Always follow the directions. Do not overuse. Start with once or twice a week to make sure your skin can tolerate them without getting red or irritated.

Consult Beaute's Expose Multi-Action Skin Polish works mechanically (with a super-fine sand) and chemically (by getting into your pores and kicking out the dirt). Unlike some exfoliators you can use it every day, which I do. I mix a tiny drop of it into our cleanser, let it sit on my face for a minute to allow the active ingredients to work, then wash it off. All exfoliants can be drying, even ours, so this method keeps my skin moist.

Never use harsh facial scrubs; your skin is not a dirty saucepan! Too much exfoliation will make your skin thinner, tighter, and more prone to irritation. It also leaves your skin looking waxy and weird.

The electric face-cleansing device with different brushes is popular but when I used it regularly my face broke out; sometimes, when you overstimulate your skin, you stir things up. My recommendation is to only use the softest brush, and use a hydrating oil-based or creamy cleanser that will make it less likely for your skin to get pulled. Or think of the device as an exfoliator—if so, only use it several times a week. If you notice any irritation or breakouts, stop using it for a couple of weeks and let your skin rest.

Since your body skin is thicker and less prone to irritation than your facial skin, you can use scrubs in the shower or bath. I also use a plastic loofa—it's much cheaper and easier to clean than a natural loofa.

Recommended Brands—Face

Chantecaille Bamboo and Hibiscus Exfoliating Cream, Consult Beaute Expose Multi-Action Skin Polish, Philosophy Resurface Microdelivery Dual-Phase Peel, Radical Skincare Age-Defying Exfoliating Pads, Sunday Riley Good Genes Treatment, Kate Somerville ExfoliKate, Konjac Facial Cleansing and Exfoliating Beauty Sponges, Ulta Nip+Fab Glycolic Fix Exfoliating Facial Pads

Recommended Brands—Face Rinse-Off Masks/Peels

Boscia Charcoal Pore Pudding, Laneige Brightening Sparkling Water Peeling Mask, Primera Peeling Facial Mild, Skin Food Black Sugar Mask, Skin Inc. Pure Revival Peel, Joanna Vargas Exfoliating Mask

Recommended Brands—Body

Kat Burki Raw Sugar Body Scrub, Ole Henriksen Rub 'n Buff Salt
Scrub, Rituals Tao Organic White Lotus and Yi Yi Ren Mild Exfoliating Body Scrub, St. Ives Fresh Skin Apricot Scrub, J.R. Watkins Natu-
rals Sugar and Shea Body Scrub (my favorite!)

Rating: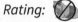

Microdermabrasion

Hype or Hot

Almost every spa uses microdermabrasion for exfoliation. The good
news is there's no recovery period. The bad news is that improvements
are minimal, so for the most part this is a waste of money.

Rating: 🚫

Lasers

Hype or Hot

The most common laser used for sluggish skin is the Fraxel, a form of
CO_2 laser. It results in minimal downtime but requires multiple treatments (three to ten) to see any kind of long-term result. I was previously a fan but over the years have come to the conclusion it's more
hype than hot. You can get better results with a good home skincare
regimen.

Rating: 🚫

Light Therapy

Hype or Hot

IPLs are designed to even out skin tones. They work if you're willing to
have dozens of them and completely stay out of the sun.

Rating:

Pore Issues

Pore-Minimizing Products

Hype or Hot

This category is often overlooked, as I don't think a lot of women know it exists. Blur products are temporary cover-ups only, acting like spackle by filling in pores and smoothing over fine lines. Just make sure the product you buy has a moisturizing agent; you don't want your face to crack when you smile! Don't expect long-term results, because enlarged pores are best treated with peels.

Recommended Brands

The Body Shop Wonderblur, Dr. Brandt Pores No More Pore Refiner Primer, Consult Beaute HD Prep Skin Perfecting Serum, Dior Pore Minimizer Skin Refining Matte Primer, Indeed Laboratories Nanoblur, Philosophy Pore Refining Duo, Smashbox Photo Finish Pore-Minimizing Foundation Primer

Rating: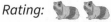

Peels

Hype or Hot

A good salicylic or glycolic acid peel can unplug dead cells from pores and help reduce the appearance of their size. A regular peel regimen can do wonders.

Rating: 🐹 🐹 🐹

Sun Damage

Sunscreen

Hype or Hot

Just so you know, an SPF of 50 isn't five times *stronger* than an SPF of 10—it just lasts longer. What matters most is UVA and UVB protection in a sunscreen that you're actually going to use properly. Physical blockers are effective but they tend to be thick, and some formulations clog your pores, causing breakouts, so test them or look for a light foundation with SPF. I keep a powder sunscreen in my purse, as it's an easy way to reapply and get rid of your shine, and it's water-resistant. They come tinted or clear, so men and children can use them, too.

Recommended Brands

Anthelios 60 Ultra Light Sunscreen Fluid, Clinique Moisture Surge CC Cream Hydrating Colour Corrector Broad Spectrum, ColoreScience Sunforgettable Mineral Sunscreen Brush, Coola Classic Sport SPF 50, Coppertone Water Babies SPF 50, Laura Mercier Tinted Moisturizer Broad Spectrum, NARS Pure Radiant Tinted Moisturizer Broad Spectrum, Tarte BB Tinted Treatment 12-Hour Primer Broad Spectrum

Rating: 🐹 🐹 🐹 🐹

Lasers

Hype or Hot

Lasers can be incredibly effective to reduce the discoloration and scattered hyper- and hypopigmentation due to sun damage. They remove the top layers of skin, rejuvenating the overall skin color and tone, and they can target the cells containing the pigment color you want diminished.

Rating: 🐹 🐹 🐹 🐹

Light Therapy

See Discoloration and Hyperpigmentation on pages 185–186

Self-Tanners

Hype or Hot

I love self-tanners—except on my face. I never use them there, since there are plenty of tinted sunscreens, moisturizers, makeup with SPF, and bronzers to use. An orange Oompa Loompa face is *not* a good look! But don't make the mistake of thinking that self-tanners will give you any sun protection—all they do is give you the color you want without sun exposure. They can't fix or hide sun damage, unless you apply tanner to try to match the color of the freckles or brown spots you got at the beach, which is a trick I'd never recommend as it's bound to go wrong!

It's hard to predict how your skin will react to a self-tanner, so plan to experiment and go slow. You can always repeat the process to get a deeper tan, but if you apply too much, you can look fake or orange. Always be sure to use a mitt or gloves so your palms don't turn a color not found in nature. Also, a salon spray-on tan can be effective—the esthetician will be able to apply it evenly all over your body. You don't want to look like a zebra!

Recommended Brands
Million Dollar Tan, Origins The Great Pretender, Suave Visible Glow, Tarte Brazilliance, Xen-Tan Sunless Tan

Rating:

Aging's Effect on Your Features—Face and Neck

Cheeks—Sagging

Firming Creams

See the Anti-Aging: Loss of Firmness and Elasticity section on page 175.

Fillers

Hype or Hot
Fillers can only add volume. They do not correct sagging!

Rating:

Lasers

See the Anti-Aging: Loss of Firmness and Elasticity section on page 175.

Facelift

Hype or Hot

The facelift is the gold standard for cheek and facial tightening. No other procedure or treatment has the potential to rejuvenate the face like a facelift. It is my absolute favorite procedure and comprises about 50 percent of my plastic surgery practice. The key is to do this procedure early and conservatively; a mini-lift in your mid-forties is easier to do and recover from, and you'll avoid that that "work done" look.

Rating:

Chin—Sagging and Jowls

Botox

Hype or Hot

Botox can be injected around your jowls to minimize them and provide lift, although the results are temporary. One of its best uses is for women who get fullness in the jaw area from masseter muscle hypertrophy that leads to a widening of the face. A small injection at the back of the jawline on each side restores that elegant narrow jawline of the younger face.

Rating:

Eyes—Sagging Upper Eyelids

Botox

Hype or Hot

Botox injected in the area just below the outer brow margin can give you a Botox brow lift, which elevates the brow and pulls upper eyelid skin with it.

Rating:

Upper Blepharoplasty

Hype or Hot

This procedure is the only other effective way to rejuvenate the upper eyelids, as it removes upper lid skin. If done properly it looks amazing and is permanent.

Rating: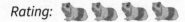

Eyes—Sagging Lower Eyelids/Under-Eye Circles

Lower Blepharoplasty

Hype or Hot

Lower eyelids are trickier and you must assess the amount of laxity or looseness of the lower eyelid muscle, but it's absolutely fantastic if you go to a skilled oculoplastic or plastic surgeon.

Rating: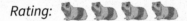

Forehead—Sagging

Botox

Hype or Hot

Injections at the outer upper eyelid can give you a "Botox brow lift," raising the brow into a more youthful position.

Rating:

Brow Lift

Hype or Hot

Because Botox can work well, and a forehead lift can be very painful, this isn't high on your list of must-do's unless your brow is descending badly.

Rating: 🐹 🐹

Lips—Thin or Uneven

Lip Plumpers

Hype or Hot

Lip plumpers work like cellulite creams—they cause irritation that slightly swells up your lips. I'm not sure they *actually* work, but I've been known to buy them anyway. That tingly sensation makes you feel plumper and juicier, but I definitely take it off before I kiss Terry!

Recommended Brands

Advanced Clinicals Collagen Instant Plumping Serum, Estée Lauder New Dimension Plump + Fill Expert Lip Treatment, Lip Service Collagen Lip Plumper, Physicians Formula Plump Potion, StriVectin Lip Plumping Treatment, Vernal Lustful Lips Plumper

Rating: 🐹 🐹

Fillers

Hype or Hot

If done properly and with a *light* touch, fillers can make lips look more feminine and can fill out deflated lips as we age. Yes, filler is abused; yes, less is more. The overinflated "trout pout" from too much lip filler is not only so *Real Housewives* but so five years ago. Start with a max of 1 cc, with half given in the upper and lower lip.

Heather: I have to admit, I like my lips. They are a nice shape and color and even though they're not perfect, I can fix the shape with my lip pencil. Would they look better with filler? Probably not, since I just hate the filler effect; no matter how subtle, it's still ducky looking. People want to see *you* walk in the room, not your lips. I also wonder once this fad fades (as they always do), what happens then? Deflated lips? That's not sexy at all.

Rating: 🐹 🐹 🐹 🐹 *when done right,* 🚫 *when overfilled*

Nose

Botox Lift

Hype or Hot

I did this to myself by injecting Botox in the tip of my nose and it was very painful. Not worth it for a tiny bit of lift that doesn't last more than a few months.

Rating: 🐹

Rhinoplasty

Hype or Hot

This will always be the one and only procedure for any changes to your nose.

Rating: 🐹 🐹 🐹 🐹

Aging's Effect on Your Features—Body

Arms—Sagging

Arm Lift

Hype or Hot

The scars are very long and the recuperation can be stressful—think about how often you move your arms every day! Recommended only after weight loss when there is a large amount of excess skin.

Rating: 🐹 🐹

Belly—Sagging and Excess Skin

Fat Dissolving

Hype or Hot

Cryolipolysis and SculpSure (see page 209 in chapter 9) are overrated!

Rating: 🐹 🐹

Liposuction

Hype or Hot

Liposuction is horrible, good, or great depending on the amount of fat you have in the area, the looseness of the skin, and the specific area you're treating. Best candidates are people with isolated fat deposits, tight skin, and areas overlying bones (love handles, outer thighs). Worst candidates are those with loose skin in areas prone to irregularities and cellulite (inner thighs, front thighs). It can also be life-changing when treating thick calves and ankles, although few surgeons have the skills to do it properly.

Rating: 🐹 🐹 🐹

Tummy Tuck

Hype or Hot

It's all about the scar. No other procedure in plastic surgery ends up with such a large scar as well as such a long recovery, yet the most impressive results and the happiest patients. If you are done having kids and you have loose skin and a belly that diet and exercise won't touch, this is the procedure for you. When choosing a doctor to perform this, look very carefully at the belly button results he shows and ask him if you will be staying overnight under nurse supervision. These two issues separate a good result from a potential disaster, as tummy tucks are the most dangerous procedures in plastic surgery. Frequent and early ambulation (walking) post-surgery go miles to prevent the most dreaded complication, the blood clot, from ruining an otherwise great procedure.

Rating: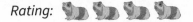

Breasts—Sagging

Temporary Breast Lift

See page 235 in chapter 9.

Rating: 🚫

Breast Lift

Hype or Hot

The breast lift will definitely lift up sagging breasts—but it will also leave scars. Very visible scars. Think long and hard before you decide to do this! And by the way, *nothing* you do in the gym can lift sagging breasts!

Rating: 🐹 🐹

Augmentation

Hype or Hot

Breast implants are great and a disaster at the same time. It's the most common plastic surgery procedure and the one that goes wrong the most. The secret is to place them under the muscle with silicone (better than saline) and don't get greedy! The body fights back when you put in a larger implant that stretches the skin. Most women look great with implants ranging from 250 (very small) to 500 cc. If you have lots of loose skin after breast-feeding, sometimes even larger makes sense. Here's a key piece of info: if you get implants you will need two or three more operations either to treat a complication or to change size as you get older and heavier. It's a commitment. If you can avoid implants and be happy, I would recommend you do!

Rating: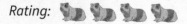

Buttocks—Shaping

Liposuction

Hype or Hot

Never, I repeat, *never* let a surgeon suction your buttock. It will loosen the skin and drop the cheeks.

Rating:

Brazilian Butt Lift

Hype or Hot

This is the hottest procedure right now and celebs are lining up for it. Generally, 300 to 900 cc are transferred to each cheek. If you have a flat buttock with little projection, it works really well. Don't get greedy, though; the more fat you transfer the greater the chance some of it will die and you can get painful lumps or infections.

Rating:

Buttock Implants

Hype or Hot

Buttock implants are effective for those with no body fat and a flat projection. Because there can be so many complications, it's a marginal procedure at best.

Rating:

Cellulite

Heather: Since cellulite has plagued me all my life, and I have tried *everything*, I have finally found that the *best* way to reduce it is with squats. Sorry, but this is true!

Rating:

Cellulite Products

Hype or Hot

No OTC product is a truly effective long-term cellulite crusher. You might get temporary relief, but don't shell out big bucks or fall for any hype. What temporarily diminishes the appearance of cellulite is increased blood flow to the area, so any form of massage with a rich cream or lotion will help.

Recommended Brands

Bodishape Cellulite Cream, Nuxe Body Lift Cellulite Serum, Oz Shape Slimming Counter Gel-Cream, Puressant Cellulite Reducing Cream, TriLASTIN-CF Cellulite Firming Complex Cream

Rating:

Endermologie

Hype or Hot

Even though this treatment gives you only temporary results, if you do it consistently you can see a dent in your cellulite. I didn't think the amount of time these treatments take and the cost are worth the limited results.

Rating: 🐹 🐹

Liposuction

Hype or Hot

Liposuction will *always* make cellulite worse. Never do it!

Rating: 🚫

Thighs—Sagging and Excess Skin

Lasers

Hype or Hot

Despite the hype, lasers don't work on sagging thighs. Save your money.

Rating: 🚫

Liposuction

Hype or Hot

Awesome for outer thighs with good skin tone, mediocre at best for inner thighs, and crummy to good in all other areas, depending on laxity of skin.

Rating: 🐹 *to* 🐹 🐹 🐹 🐹 *depending on skin and area*

◇◇◇◇◇◇◇◇◇◇◇◇◇◇◇◇◇◇◇◇

Take it from Dr. and Mrs. Guinea Pig, we've tried it all so you don't have to, and we hope this chapter will become your quick reference guide for the good, the bad, and the ugly when it comes to skincare products and procedures. Next up, the hippest, hottest, newest . . . buyer beware!

PART
IV

The Good, the Bad, and the Crazy

CHAPTER
9

Hippest, Hottest, Newest—What Works and What Doesn't

We live in Southern California, which is often thought of as the epicenter of not just geologic faults but every crazy new kind of skincare treatment anyone can possibly subject themselves to. Hippest, hottest, newest—it's all here in Hollywood. For better or for worse, we are inundated with the latest and greatest (or not) that the rich and famous have to offer.

We listed and rated the most common and well-tested anti-aging treatments in the previous part of this book, but here we are detailing the most out-there. We hear about them through the grapevine, which is always groaning under the weight of "I heard so-and-so is doing such and such . . ." We get pitched by hyperbole-drenched public relations companies. We follow social media sites that breathlessly report on new trends in beauty and health. And guess what? Some of the hippest, hottest, newest treatments, we're happy to report, actually work! Most of them, however, are extremely effective only for the charlatan hyping the treatment and taking your hard-earned money for it.

A word of advice: We know how much you want to dunk your heads in the fountain of youth for an endless drink. We are happy to be Dr. and Mrs. Guinea Pig for all the treatments in this chapter—but we also want to warn you that you really, really want to avoid the newest of the new. When our computer software is about to be upgraded, our techies always tell us to wait a while so the bugs get worked out first. Wise words—and you should follow them about all skincare treatments, too! So let *us* be your guides, your testers, your guinea pigs.

Note: Heather wrote about the noninvasive treatments, and Terry wrote about the medical ones, unless otherwise specified.

Acupuncture Facelift

What It Does

Allegedly tightens the skin of your face.

How It Works

Super-fine acupuncture needles are inserted at various pressure points in your face. A few others may be inserted at other points in your body.

Lasts For

As long as you think it does!

Possible Complications

None.

Avoid Being Botched

Go only to an experienced and licensed therapist. Acupuncture shouldn't hurt, but sometimes when a needle is placed in a particular point (especially on the feet), there is a sharp twinge that lasts for about a second.

Science or Scary

Chinese medicine and acupuncture have been in use for thousands of years. Acupuncture has been extensively studied and we believe it does have an effect on certain conditions, such as pain relief and improving the overall health of your immune system. When I was trying to have a baby, I couldn't get pregnant so we did in vitro fertilization, and I had a lot of acupuncture until my babies were born. I was willing to try absolutely anything. There's something to be said for lying there in a dark room with a treatment that improves your overall circulation. So, while you can't tighten your skin by putting needles in your face, you can improve the overall health of your skin. And you can certainly feel a lot better. And if a treatment makes you feel better, you *will* look better!

At-Home Devices

One of the newest trends in the anti-aging business is the development of devices you can use in the privacy of your own bathroom—devices intended to replace the powerful machines dermatologists and plastic surgeons use in their offices. Are they worth it? It's hard to do due diligence online, as most of the testimonial pages that have actual people posting are evenly split between true believers and complete skeptics!

IPL/LED Light Therapy Devices

What It Does

When used at home, it might reduce your wrinkles and acne, but it also might burn the skin right off you.

How It Works

During a professional treatment, a sensitizing agent applied to the skin is activated by the light, causing what is basically a controlled sunburn. At home, only the light is used, removing much of the effectiveness but maintaining the risk of complications.

Lasts For

If it does work on your acne, then your acne will diminish with regular use.

Possible Complications

Intense pain, burning, itching, redness, blisters, crusting, skin infections.

Avoid Being Botched

Let a doctor do it. The light might kill some of the acne that causes bacteria, but OTC treatments are effective, especially if you follow my treatment plan on page 171.

Science or Scary

Science if performed properly; scary if not.

Lasers for Hair Removal

What It Does

Destroys hair follicles so hair doesn't grow back.

How It Works

Using a concentrated light, hair follicles growing in the target area are zapped into oblivion and cannot regrow themselves.

Lasts For

If it works, it's supposedly permanent. As you know, though, hair doesn't grow evenly and follicles are in different stages of rest/growth, so repeated treatments over a period of time will always be needed. *Heather:* I found this treatment very effective for legs and underarms, but it takes a *long* time to do the treatment, and because of hair growth cycles you need four to six treatments per area.

Possible Complications

Some people can't bear the pain of the prickly feeling, although it is minimal, and the newest lasers boast a pain-free experience. Otherwise, there isn't much risk due to the power of the laser being significantly downgraded from the one used by medical professionals.

Avoid Being Botched

Take it easy on yourself, or just get a doctor to do it.

Science or Scary

There are many different hair removers on the market and they are very popular, as consumers can control the intensity and take their time doing their treatments. It's definitely worth it in the long run, but difficult to keep going.

Lasers for Wrinkle Reduction

What It Does

The laser is meant to spur new collagen growth and lessen the appearance of wrinkles.

How It Works

As with a professional laser, a concentrated beam of light is directed onto your skin.

Lasts For

Unknown—everyone will react differently, but mostly when you get a wrinkle- reduction result it tends to be permanent.

Possible Complications

Pain (like lots of tiny needles prickling your face), burning, swelling, reddened skin.

Avoid Being Botched

Again, let a doctor perform this potentially dangerous procedure.

Science or Scary

Lasers work—when wielded by competent, well-trained medical professionals. An at-home device is basically ineffective, so don't bother.

Cryolipolysis and SculpSure

What It Does

Reduces fat in a non-invasive procedure.

How It Works

Cryolipolysis uses cold and SculpSure uses heat to deliberately injure fat cells, and when they die your body excretes them, diminishing fat.

Lasts For

Once the fat is destroyed using either of these devices the results are permanent, provided you keep your weight stable.

Possible Complications

Soreness and swelling after the procedure, but it is relatively painless and requires no downtime afterward. Blisters and hyperpigmentation have been reported, as well as prolonged burning pain called neuralgia.

Avoid Being Botched

Make sure you seek out the latest device, because earlier models had a higher complication rate.

Science or Scary

These devices are FDA-approved for the abdomen and flanks only, but they can be used off-label in any area of concern. Some patients are pleased with the outcome, but it's not liposuction—a 30 to 40 percent improvement is the most you can expect, if that. Also, these devices are super hyped and getting complaints for little improvement. Don't do it if your skin is loose, as it will just loosen the skin further. Frankly, a good diet is more effective.

Cosmetic Medicine

This category includes different prescription medications and stem cell therapies that should be obtained only through consultations and visits to a specialist physician.

Hormone Replacement Therapy—Estrogen and Progesterone for Women and Testosterone for Men

What It Does

Hormone replacement therapy (HRT) is a form of supplementation given when the female (estrogen and progesterone) and male (testosterone) hormones naturally begin to decline with age. For women, this is usually in their forties; for men, it could be their thirties or forties.

How It Works

Supplements restore hormone levels. You want to take a level that brings you back to what was normal to you in your twenties or thirties; no more or no less. What I would recommend you consider is restoring your hormone levels to approximately how they were when you weren't fatigued, you felt strong and healthy, and your sexual energy was appropriate.

For women, HRT can be either pills, vaginal inserts, or bioidentical creams that are applied to the inner thighs. For men, testosterone is usually given transdermally, with a gel that comes in a pump device and is applied with the fingers to the chest and shoulders.

Lasts For

As long as you keep taking it.

Possible Complications

For women, there have been studies showing a very slightly elevated risk of strokes and heart disease with long-term HRT. Discuss your health concerns with your gynecologist. Most women decide that a low dose is worth any risks, since it alleviates such symptoms as weight gain, moodiness, brain fog, hot flashes, lower energy, loss of libido, bone loss, drier skin and hair, and insomnia that are affecting their daily lives. Ditto for men, who might be dealing with a loss of libido, loss of muscle mass, fatigue, or lower energy. For men, if the dose is too high, the side effects are nasty: mood disorders, especially a propensity to anger; thinning hair; man boobs; smaller testicles; and acne, especially on the back and buttocks.

Avoid Being Botched

Start with the lowest possible dose that relieves your symptoms. Have your hormone levels tested regularly by your gynecologist or urologist. Report any unusual symptoms.

Science or Scary

The best kind of science. I am very much in favor of HRT, and I think we're about five to ten years away from saying that men need to go on HRT just like women. I've seen how many of my patients have benefitted from it, so don't be shy about discussing your needs with your doctor!

Human Growth Hormone

What It Does

In terms of pure cosmetic medicine, human growth hormone increases your muscle mass to make you look more fit and ripped. It makes you stronger, it makes you feel faster, it lessens your recovery times when you work out or you have an injury. You have more energy and you sleep better.

There is no question that HGH makes a very youthful appearance, with a better skin tone and thicker hair. It erases wrinkles, too. If I haven't seen friends who've been on HGH for more than six months and then they walk into my office, they'll look unnaturally youthful in a good way. They get the *glow.* They look like actors and celebrities who are extraordinarily blessed genetically. They just look better than the rest of us.

How It Works

HGH decreases your overall body fat composition while it increases your lean muscle mass, which is why professional athletes take it on the sly—and why, of course, it's banned. They're not going to fool around with getting kicked out of their sport unless whatever they're sneaking will truly give them an edge. Let's face it, they're using growth hormone because it makes them look and feel better, and be better athletes. No one can yet pinpoint precisely how it affects skin, but it's obviously through cell regeneration processes.

Lasts For

Forever. But only if you keep getting the injections. The amount varies depending on your goals, but generally speaking you need three to seven IU (international units) done three to five times week. Got that? Shots practically every other day. As soon as you stop, the effects start to wear off. My general rule with anti-aging medications, as with diet and exercise, is that it takes half the time you took the drug to get the effect to lose it. In other words, if you were on HGH for six months, all the effects would be gone within three months of you stop taking it.

I expect that someday it will be possible to use a transdermal patch for HGH, as is done for testosterone. My general vibe is that when people say, "There will never be a way to XYX," then, on the contrary, there will always be a way to XYZ. It just takes time. Once I laid my eyes on the very first generation of iPhones, I knew this was a new world. I firmly believed that anything was possible—and I still do!

Possible Complications

One is joint pain, often in the wrists, which can lead to carpel tunnel syndrome. If you're taking metformin for your glucose levels, it can also, theoretically, expose your cells to greater oxidation side effects, creating a higher cancer risk. The other complications are to your bank account (it is *very* expensive and never covered by insurance unless you have true HGH deficiency, which is very rare) and the time factor for shots at least three times a week. Most people who take it learn to self-inject.

Avoid Being Botched

There are tons of topical products and supplements designed to increase your natural HGH levels. They do *not* work. You absolutely *cannot* ingest a growth hormone releasing factor or a direct HGH that will be metabolized so it can be effective. The only way to increase HGH levels is through injection with a needle. In addition, there is a lot of black market HGH out there due to its cost, but that is extremely risky and no one should be dumb enough to buy it.

Science or Scary

I would recommend considering HGH for anyone who is a senior (age sixty-five and over) and in good health yet who's reached a stage in their life where their skin is showing easy bruising, they've got aches and pains, and they've suddenly gotten *old*. Like a craggy old version of themselves. They've lost that *sparkle*. That sparkle is exactly what HGH growth hormone gives you back.

Would I recommend it for someone in their forties or even fifties who's trying to push back the clock? Absolutely not.

One of the problems with HGH is that it's not one of these things like diet and exercise where you do look a lot better after a lot of hard work. HGH is more subtle, and it takes at least six to nine months before that glow starts to appear. After a certain age, though, if you want to look the best version of yourself, you use everything at your disposal if you understand the risks. HGH is one of those things. Yes, it might not be safe because it hasn't been out on the market for very long, and it may increase your risk of getting cancer. But if you're seventy-two and already at a higher cancer risk due solely to your age, HGH is simply something to consider. And guess what—cosmetic surgery isn't safe and we do know what the risks are. You can die from cosmetic surgery and get infections and scars and other complications.

So to me it's all part of the same melting pot of ways to prolong your life, look better, and stay youthful. I don't "recommend" cosmetic surgery in the same way I don't "recommend" HGH. These are elective treatments that are effective and that can be used very safely under the proper guidance.

Metformin

What It Does

As you likely know, excess consumption of sugar is very aging, and it also puts you at a higher risk for obesity, diabetes, and cancer. Studies with animals now are showing that metformin is prolonging their life span and making them less susceptible to tumors and plaque buildup in their arteries.

How It Works

This medication is often used for weight management, as it makes you less sensitive to insulin, and it affects the absorption of glucose in cells.

Lasts For

Theoretically, as long as you keep taking it.

Possible Complications

There might be low-level gastrointestinal problems such as bloating or diarrhea. Some people get mild headaches. Start at a low level. One of the best side effects is weight loss!

Avoid Being Botched

Have a thorough physical before starting and regular appointments afterward to monitor your blood sugar.

Science or Scary

Definitely science. Metformin is one of the most exciting new frontiers in anti-aging, as it's thought to help cells live longer—which is what slows down the entire aging process. I refer to it as one of the ingredients in the Doctor Cocktail that so many physicians are on now (along with HGH and testosterone, if they're male), and they all look great, with glowing skin and increased energy levels. I'm not on it since the jury's still out, but it's thrilling to follow the ongoing research and hope that someday this kind of drug will help us live a longer life with a lower chance of heart disease.

Stem Cell Therapy

What It Does

Stem cells are the cells in your body that have the potential to form into any kind of specific cell that you would need in an area where you're trying to affect a positive outcome. They supposedly have growth factors and compounds in them to allow for faster healing.

How It Works

It doesn't.

Lasts For

It doesn't last because it never worked in the first place!

Possible Complications

None. Except you throwing money out the window.

Avoid Being Botched

Save your money for other, more effective treatments! People are being ripped off and paying extraordinary amounts of money for very expensive snake oil.

Science or Scary

"Stem cells" is one of those wastebasket categories of terms where it's easy to imply magical powers, and at this point it's incredibly exaggerated, overused, and has very, very limited ability to do anything. Some people claim that if you add stem cells to fat transfers it will prevent fat re-absorption, but there is no scientific evidence for that, either.

Cryotherapy

What It Does

Cryotherapy is the use of extreme cold in any kind of medical treatment. What people hope it does for anti-aging is improve circulation, strengthen the immune system, increase collagen production, and maybe even make a dent in cellulite.

How It Works

You go into a chamber, wearing nothing more than light clothing and socks and gloves or mitts on your hands and nose to prevent frostbite injury, and you are blasted with liquid nitrogen–cooled air down to about −40 degrees for about three minutes. Most people have sessions once or twice a week for several weeks.

Lasts For

There are perhaps some positive benefits, but they're hard to measure, and that's especially so for skin. More sessions are not going to give you better results.

Possible Complications

Frostbite, if you are in the machine too long and your extremities aren't protected. Death, if the machine malfunctions. A woman who worked at a cryotherapy salon was killed in 2015 when she decided to give herself a treatment after hours and somehow got locked in the machine. She froze to death in minutes.

Avoid Being Botched

If you've got arthritis, aches, pains, fatigue, or an illness and you want to try this for a few weeks to see if these conditions improve, or if you're doing it for general rejuvenating properties, you don't need to go more than once a week for six weeks. Or, you could stay home and enjoy a cold shower!

Science or Scary

Thirty years ago, when I was a medical student, if you had told me that when someone's in a dramatic accident and has a bad injury, the staff in the ER would freeze them down in a severely hypothermic state, put them in a coma, and stop all the inflammatory and injury process, I would have frozen in my steps and thought you were nuts! But here we are—now when patients have a catastrophic brain injury or heart attack, they often get brought to the hospital and we freeze them down.

It's pretty clear now that even in traditional medicine we appreciate the powerful effects of cryotherapy on our bodies. Athletes use it all the time—even with something as simple as an ice bath—to reduce inflammation in sore muscles.

But for your skin, or for rejuvenation? Please don't waste your time!

Crystal Therapy

What It Does

Uses the placement of different crystals to alter the user's energy flow to prevent or cure disease.

How It Works

For those who believe that crystals have energetic qualities, using them can allegedly improve energy and circulation. For those who don't believe, putting crystals on your skin does absolutely nothing—but if you like the idea of being surrounded by gems, maybe it's better to visit Tiffany or Cartier!

Lasts For

Can you prove scientifically that crystal therapy has any effect? No.

Possible Complications

Unless you encounter a particularly jagged crystal, none.

Avoid Being Botched

Some crystals are very expensive. Shop around!

Science or Scary

Terry: Yes, I know it can be scary that people sometimes put more faith in rocks than doctors, but I am a practicing Buddhist and I believe in the power of centering as one with the elements. Like acupuncture for the Chinese, crystals are part of many ancient traditions for a reason that is not just spiritually symbolic. They have some sort of essence to them. Warriors made them into talismans and wore them into battle. Scoff if you like, but I feel better knowing that my crystals are near me at work and at home. So while crystals can't be proven to provide any anti-aging benefits, for me they fall into the category of "if it does no harm, no harm in doing it." They're sort of like the placebo effect, which I discussed in chapter 6—potentially an objective, powerful thing because it uses a mystical, mysterious force we don't understand to make a very real mind/body connection.

Drinkable Collagen

What It Does

Drinking collagen will support collagen growth everywhere in your body and improve the appearance of your skin.

How It Works

It used to be impossible to metabolize collagen when ingested because it would be destroyed by stomach acids. We developed our Beaute Shot Cocktail with two kinds of hydrolyzed collagen that *can* be absorbed; it also includes ceramides, which are proteins that work with cells at the cell membrane level to reduce micro-wrinkling. This increases the level of moisture in your skin and diminishes the appearance of roughness. Our drinkable collagen comes as a liquid, and you can add it to anything hot or cold, such as your tea or a smoothie. This is truly drinkable skincare!

Lasts For

As long as you keep drinking it. If you really want to improve your collagen, think of this drink as akin to diet and exercise—you sort of need to do it every day.

Possible Complications

None.

Avoid Being Botched

You already know that collagen molecules are too big to pass through skin. If you want to ingest collagen, make sure that whatever you're using actually can get absorbed by your body. Buy it from a reliable source!

Science or Scary

The very best science—because we've seen the data. Now you can treat your skin from the inside out as well as the outside in. Our Beaute Shake is a meal-replacement shake that is dairy-free, gluten-free, sugar-free, lactose-free, and loaded with antioxidants in the form of superfruit extracts, and each serving is only 100 calories. Plus it has collagen and hyaluronic acid to support beautiful, youthful skin. It's not only super filling—it's really good for you.

Electrostimulation

What It Does

If the claims are to be believed, it improves skin cell turnover and stimulates cell growth, helps you sleep, and reduces stress. If you have an actual muscular injury, it may help with the pain a bit.

How It Works

Electrodes are placed on the skin, and a current is sent from one to the other, stimulating the parts of the body in between.

Lasts For

Unclear, if at all. A lot of salons that offer it say you need multiple treatments, which always makes me very wary!

Possible Complications

These machines have been around for years so at least you know you're not going to get electrocuted. The tiny bit of current isn't harmful, even if it isn't particularly beneficial.

Avoid Being Botched

Don't do it if the source of the electricity is any larger than a handheld device. Also, make sure that the person doing this has a clue, as you don't want it turned up to the highest level, just in case.

Science or Scary

Electrostimulation is the epitome of scary science, like Frankenstein. It doesn't work, and it's one of those kind of hocus-pocus treatments, usually added on to a facial, where you think it's going to do something because you can *feel* it. Yes, it might well increase the blood flow to your face, but you can do that at home by rubbing your skin.

Facials

I love facials and get them regularly. They can improve hydration, clear up blemishes, or even out your skin tone. Still, facials are really about improving the blood flow to your skin, putting you in a wonderful state of relaxation, and providing a deep cleaning and exfoliation so your regular products will work more effectively.

Would you know that from some of the facials listed here? No, you would not! Be sure to ask how long the treatment is, its specific services, the products used, and the cost.

Above all, make sure your esthetician is well trained and licensed, and understands skin. Many of them do not. This is a good time to read online reviews (carefully overlooking the ones the technician's friends and family members are posting for them!). I've had friends walk out of facials looking worse, with tight and blotchy skin and red marks from overzealous extractions of whiteheads and pimples. Or even bruised and broken out. The rule of thumb is that you should walk out of a facial looking better than when you went in. Even without makeup!

Blood Facial

What It Does

It's touted to give you a youthful glow as well as tighten your skin.

How It Works

Allegedly, your own blood is rich with stem cells and growth factors that will penetrate into your skin to rejuvenate it. After your blood is drawn, it's centrifuged so that only platelet-rich plasma (full of red blood cells) can be applied to your face.

Lasts For

No time at all, because it's bogus.

Possible Complications

None, other than having any problems with the blood draw, such as an infection.

Avoid Being Botched

Don't even think about wasting your time on this.

Science or Scary

A blood facial is hyped as helping rejuvenate your skin, but there are no HGH factors floating around in your bloodstream, and even if there were, they couldn't penetrate into your skin when applied in a facial. Blood isn't exactly high on the list of super-hydrating fluids! This is nothing more than vampire BS.

Caviar/Truffle Facial

What It Does

Luxury food items are placed on your face and the nutrients are allegedly absorbed through the skin, fighting aging and providing a glow.

How It Works

It doesn't, because nutrients from food are absorbed through the stomach, not the skin.

Lasts For

Until you get hungry. But the pungent odors can linger long afterward in your nose!

Possible Complications

If you're spending hundreds of dollars on the most expensive foods in the world and rubbing them on your skin instead of devouring them, you've probably gone insane. Also, people will avoid you because of the stench on your face! Other than that, none.

Avoid Being Botched

Go out to dinner instead.

Science or Scary

Scary that these people are willing to spend so much money on this waste of delicious food. They should at least demand a glass of champs, too!

Gold Facial

What It Does

Claims to improve skin's texture, tone, appearance, redness, elasticity, wrinkles, dark spots, and hydration. Did you hear that even Cleopatra used it?

How It Works

Once a gold scrub is applied and massaged in, sheets of gold foil are stuck to the skin. This reportedly can penetrate the skin to create a golden glow. Except, of course, this doesn't happen at all because gold can't get into or through your skin.

Lasts For

Until you wash it off and watch hundreds of dollars' worth of gold flow down the drain.

Possible Complications

Some may develop an allergy to gold as a result of repeated treatment.

Avoid Being Botched

Because gold is pretty safe for humans (that's why it's used in dental fillings), there isn't much risk.

Science or Scary

Scary how a celebrity endorsement of a luxury item is seen as scientific evidence by many.

Oxygen Facial

What It Does

When performed at a spa, the practitioner uses a device that blows high levels of almost pure oxygen all over a previously treated face, supposedly improving its absorption to rejuvenate skin.

How It Works

If you believe that skin gets asphyxiated and needs a directed gust of pure oxygen to breathe, then it works by adding a dose of the placebo effect to your spa experience.

Lasts For

Until you go outside, feel the wind on your face, and realize you will never get your time or money back.

Possible Complications

It can't harm you. Except you can feel really dumb for thinking that just because oxygen is necessary to survive it doesn't mean that using it for skincare would be a good idea.

Avoid Being Botched

Take a deep breath.

Science or Scary

Scary how the word "oxygen" is esoteric enough that people are still buying into this. Oxygen facials are very popular, but they have *not* been proven to increase cell turnover or rejuvenate your skin in a significant way. Terry doesn't believe in the power of delivering high levels of oxygen to the skin during a facial, and you shouldn't either.

Placenta Facial

What It Does

It claims to fight aging, provide a healthful glow, repair damaged skin, and cure all diseases.

How It Works

Thankfully, it is only a placenta extract that is being used. Apparently, the stem cells in the placenta contain anti-aging properties, which proponents claim will be absorbed through the skin despite the fact that's not at all how stem cells work.

Lasts For

As long as the treatment would have without the added placenta.

Possible Complications

None, apart from being grossed out by the fact that a part of a sheep's placenta is now on your face.

Avoid Being Botched

Don't try it at home.

Science or Scary

It's scary how people can be convinced that something is scientific because the phrase "stem cell" is involved.

Snail Slime Facial

What It Does

Snail slime is meant to even out your skin tone and revitalize your complexion. Some claims are made that it helps reduce acne, too.

How It Works

Snail slime, or mucin, contains enzymes, sugars, and even a bit of hyaluronic acid. Allegedly, these components will have an effect on skin. Note the use of the word *allegedly*.

Lasts For

It depends. Snail slime is found in many different products in South Korea, and they're very popular. Some people like this ingredient and feel it gives their skin a glow.

Possible Complications

You could be allergic to or get irritated by the slime.

Avoid Being Botched

There shouldn't be any problems with this ingredient when used in a facial. It's usually mixed with other moisturizing ingredients.

Science or Scary

Frankly, if you want a facial with the plumping effect of hyaluronic acid, you can get one with higher concentrations than found in snail mucus.

For plumping, I have a better idea: go eat sushi. Trip out on your soy sauce and the next day you will have that plump effect, because the high salt content in soy sauce makes you retain water, not just in your belly area but all over. When I have an event coming up and I have dropped a pound or two, my face gets a little hollow. My trick is to go for sushi the night before. It always makes my face look better.

Fake Botox

What It Does

It's touted as the real Botox, which is a neurotransmitter inhibiter; in other words, it's designed to block the connection between the neurotransmitter and the receptor at the muscle.

How It Works

If it's real, it "freezes" the muscle, as you know, which smoothes out and prevents more wrinkles from forming.

Lasts For

Several months.

Possible Complications

Botox is a relative of the kind of toxin put on the tips of blow darts to paralyze people and stop them from being able to breathe. The difference is Botox is highly diluted and only acts locally where it's injected. So with fake Botox, it's not that it's fraudulent or that it's ineffective—it's potentially lethal.

People *have* died from Botox. Not from normal and regulated cosmetic use, but from off-label use to treat migraines or neck pain. Or from quacks. There are several potential problems here, including that these substances are unregulated; they may come from really strange bacteria; they may be unpurified; and they can be adulterated with viruses and bacteria and can be incredibly dangerous.

Avoid Being Botched

Never, ever have Botox injected by anyone other than a board-certified cosmetic dermatologist or plastic surgeon, and certainly never by anyone not in a medical setting.

Science or Scary

There are fake versions of Botox made in different countries that do bind to the muscle receptor and, allegedly, work. The science is sound. The method and delivery is *not*.

By the way, it is hoped that someday there will be a topical version of Botox, and that would be a great idea. Because Botox only acts locally, it won't be able to track down to your diaphragm and stop your ability to breathe. Not that I wouldn't trust some people to think that if a little works, a lot would work even better! That's not what happens, of course. You may think two pain pills are good for your headache, but fifty will kill your liver (and you, too).

IV Beauty Infusions

What It Does

Delivers nutrients to your bloodstream directly through an IV hookup.

How It Works

A needle is placed in your vein and the ingredients from the IV pouch filter into your body and, allegedly, get more effectively to your skin cells.

Lasts For

It doesn't, because it's bogus.

Possible Complications

I find it scary that consumers are being sold on the "fact" that they're getting a high- dose concentration of nutrients and vitamins intravenously, while ignoring the fact that the complications of an IV can be very significant. You can get a superficial phlebitis, which is infection of the actual vein. That can evolve into a deep vein thrombosis, which can send a blood clot to your heart and kill you.

Avoid Being Botched

By eating a good, healthy diet and taking supplements in pill form made by a reputable manufacturer.

Science or Scary

Basically, you're paying to have an IV of things you could just as easily ingest. It certainly sounds more scientific and like you'll get more out of it because you're sticking the ingredients directly into the vein, but that's just not true.

Leech Therapy

What It Does

The leeches allegedly suck out impurities, and their saliva and juices when mixed with your blood are supposed to give you an even better tightening, anti-aging, rejuvenating effect.

How It Works

Leeches are applied to your abdominal area, and they suck your blood until they're engorged. Your blood is then "milked" out of them and applied to your skin like a mask for about thirty minutes.

Lasts For

A few hours or maybe a day or two.

Possible Complications

Leeches have a particular type of difficult-to-treat bacteria in their mouth, and if you get an infection from that, it's pretty nasty. The amount of blood taken is actually small, so you're not at risk for anemia. But this procedure really hurts, and it requires a very significant recovery period. After we tried this, Terry was in pain for *months* when he was on the treadmill at the gym, and we both had scars for over eight months. Plus, we thought the bleeding would stop right away, yet we were drenched for eight hours. We were given maxi pads (!) to duct-tape to our bellies and figured that would do the trick, as we had to go to a "bondage" party for *Real Housewives of Orange County* (that was being filmed, of course) right after we had the treatment. So we were at the party and all of a sudden I looked at Terry and saw blood dripping down his arm. Then I looked down and the entire side of my skirt was soaked in blood. We ran to the bathroom and thank goodness my friend Tamra had brought an extra dress with her. We cleaned ourselves up and luckily there was plenty of duct tape around since it was a bondage party, but it was a mess!

Avoid Being Botched

By looking at leeches in a nature documentary and not on your belly.

Science or Scary

Leeches are regularly used in medical procedures and for injuries and wounds, where they can be very effective as an anticoagulant with wound cleaning and healing. But that has nothing to do with rejuvenation. I thought my skin looked and felt light and bright afterward, but considering the pain and scarring, it wasn't worth it. And there is no proof that there are any regenerative properties in leech saliva when mixed with your blood that enhances the growth factors or any other kind of effectiveness on the skin.

Mesotherapy

What It Does

Reduces cellulite with targeted injections of different detergents and agents into the cellulite areas. The Brazilian technique uses a needle to dislodge the fibrous bands holding the cellulite in place. With Kybella, an FDA-approved form of mesotherapy for the treatment of fat cells in the jaw/double chins, injections are placed in the chin area.

How It Works

The fluid is injected underneath the skin and is designed to cause an inflammatory reaction that will potentially improve the appearance of cellulite areas or disrupt/kill fat cells.

Lasts For

Mesotherapy will seem to work for a few weeks or months since it causes a lot of local swelling, which might seem to minimize cellulite. Kybella necessitates multiple treatments, and there's no way yet to predict how well it will work or last.

Possible Complications

For cellulite, I had mesotherapy and the Brazilian technique, and it *really* hurt. I was so nauseous afterward I needed prescription meds to control it. There was also bruising, swelling, and itchiness. With Kybella, which causes inflammation that's designed to kill tissue—fat cells in particular, which are then excreted in your urine—this leads to a lot of local swelling, irritation, and redness as well as tenderness and pain for anywhere from two days to two weeks. You can also get a nodularity of cells that have died but are not cleared out and cause local granuloma processes, which are foreign body reactions that lead to scarring inside. And if any mesotherapy injections aren't done properly, they can kill the skin itself.

Avoid Being Botched

This is an unregulated treatment for cellulite, so there's no way you will be told what's actually in the injections, so there's a high risk of having a reaction, allergic or otherwise. With Kybella, only go to a cosmetic dermatologist or plastic surgeon for the treatment.

Science or Scary

Heather: I went to the only guy in town who was doing the treatments for cellulite—which right off the bat should have warned me away. Mesotherapy can have some limited effectiveness, but because it's so unclear about which injections actually work and for whom, we don't recommend it. It can be dangerous. The only thing that lessened my cellulite, as you know, was by going to the gym and doing *squats*.

Although it's more invasive than injecting Kybella, the best and easiest way to get rid of isolated fat is to do a little liposuction. It's not appropriate to use Kybella in a large area such as your abdomen or outer thigh, as it's so weak and relatively unpredictable. It would be a waste of your money and could cause the complications noted above.

Micro-Needling

What It Does

Micro-needling is an adjunct to other procedures, such as a facial, to allow for more effective penetration of the active ingredients in whatever you're putting on your skin.

How It Works

A device, usually in the form of a roller studded with tiny needles, creates micro-fissures in your skin.

Lasts For

As long as the products you're using do.

Possible Complications

None, really, unless an overzealous practitioner has a heavy hand and you bleed too much. Or you overdo it with an at-home device. It can hurt, too, so ask for numbing cream beforehand.

Avoid Being Botched

Don't try this at home. Go to an experienced doctor. There are at-home micro-needling devices, and you can actually create wounds and skin damage with repeated use.

Science or Scary

This is an effective procedure when done judiciously. Micro-needling is an excellent treatment for scar reduction, and it allows better penetration for topical treatments. It can't, however, reduce wrinkles or get rid of cellulite, so don't believe any hype if that's being touted to you.

Nonsurgical "Filler Facelift"

What It Does

Tightens your skin and/or increases the volume of the soft tissue in your face to make you look younger.

How It Works

A nonsurgical facelift is nothing more than a trick kind of term for all treatments involving fillers, lasers, or radiofrequency tightening that mimic, on a lower scale, the effects of a surgical facelift.

Lasts For

Several months to several years.

Possible Complications

See chapter 5!

Avoid Being Botched

Only go to a board-certified cosmetic dermatologist or plastic surgeon.

Science or Scary

These treatments are all based on science and they all work. But let's call a nonsurgical facelift what it is—*not* a facelift!

Rubber Sheet Masks

What It Does

Smoothes and firms skin, and removes blackheads.

How It Works

Usually sold as a DIY kit to mix and apply. Once you're done mixing the powder with water, you apply it to your face for a few minutes, then peel it off.

Lasts For

A few days, perhaps.

Possible Complications

None, if used properly.

Avoid Being Botched

There's not much downside to this mask, as it's hydrating. Just don't leave it on longer than instructed.

Science or Scary

It makes you look plenty scary when you have it on, but don't knock the therapeutic value of masks. Sheet masks are all the rage in South Korea, where skincare borders on the obsessive, and many of them target different skin issues like extreme dryness or exfoliation. What I like about the rubber masks is that they're so much fun. They come in a little cup that looks like ones of those cups of noodles, which encourages teens with blemishes or grown-ups who need hydration to use them—and that's always a good thing. Start your preteens on good skincare and it will last a lifetime!

Seaweed Wraps

What It Does

It apparently hydrates, firms, refreshes, purifies, and revitalizes the skin.

How It Works

By putting wet seaweed on your face and/or body for anywhere from fifteen minutes to over an hour, all the goodness of the sea will be conveyed into your skin. Or not, according to discrepant accounts. Seaweed is indeed a nutritious substance. Too bad you need to eat it in order to absorb those nutrients.

Lasts For

As long as you can convince yourself that putting wet seaweed on your face is better than simply washing your face.

Possible Complications

None, unless you have a seaweed allergy.

Avoid Being Botched

Don't use the wasabi-flavored kind.

Science or Scary

Scary because what will happen to our sushi if everyone decides to use all the seaweed for their faces? Kidding aside, a seaweed facial or wrap is a quick fix that's relaxing (as long as you can tolerate the briny odor) and hydrating. If you get this kind of wrap or facial at a spa, you'll get seaweed rubbed all over you and then you'll get wrapped up in foil or plastic so you're like an enormous sushi roll, and placed under a warmer so you can "cook." When you're done, you wash everything off. I like this treatment because you stay wet the entire time, and I don't believe in any kind of wrap or facial that's drying—or in any kind of treatment that's painful and then nothing happens. Afterward, my skin feels smooth and soft, but it would feel like that if I'd had oils or moisturizing creams rubbed into me and I got rolled up and baked for a short time, too. It makes me feel good—and that's really the best reason to get a wrap or any other kind of spa treatment. C'mon, guys, you know what I always say, so repeat after me: When you feel good, you look good!

Silicone, a.k.a. Pumping Parties

What It Does

Someone with something in a syringe injects it into your face or body outside a licensed medical establishment.

How It Works

Same as any injections.

Lasts For

It could be totally inert and do nothing and last for no time at all, or it could be industrial-grade silicone which lasts forever.

Possible Complications

Anything from low-level infections from the needles to flesh-eating bacteria to permanent disfigurement to death. Is that scary enough to convince you to stay away from this sort of thing? *Death!* Bogus or industrial silicone can cause a very severe reaction in your skin, where the silicone gets walled off and forms what we call granulomas, or foreign body masses. These can get infected, and once they do, they're incredibly hard to treat because they've been walled off and are not accessible to the vascular systems of the body. If they *do* get into your vascular system, they can cause pulmonary embolisms, or blood clots in the lungs, that can kill you. As for pain, micro-droplet silicone injections in the face only hurt a little, but if you're going to one of these pumping parties, they *really* hurt—but people tolerate them because they're willing to undergo a lot of pain in order to look better. Or, have severe complications and, you know, *die.*

Avoid Being Botched

Never, *ever* even think of getting "pumped." You might think you're saving money or time, but the cost to your health and pocketbook could very well be permanently catastrophic.

Science or Scary

On *Botched*, we saw a lovely transgender lady named Rajee who had made the extremely bad decision to see an unlicensed quack (who is now, mercifully, in prison) for silicone injections. She was injected with industrial-grade silicone—a caulking material that basically turned into concrete in her body—and she became severely disfigured. Although we at first turned her down for fear of causing facial paralysis, we ultimately did fix her—but it took seven different, very complex, and potentially dangerous procedures. In addition, her breasts had become so enormous and leaden that they sagged down to her abdomen, but the only way to fix them was with a double mastectomy, which she declined.

So why do so many people go to pumping parties? The problem is, when your friend, whom you know and trust, says, "Oh, well, I know the guy that does this. He's a doctor. Look at my face, look how amazing I look, he's the *best*!" You trust your friend and you don't vet the alleged pumper. Are you going to do a background check? No. But this is a risk no one should ever take!

Temporary Breast Lift

What It Does
Temporarily increases the size of your breasts so you can see how you'd look with a breast augmentation.

How It Works
Sterile saline is injected into your breasts.

Lasts For
About twenty-four hours, maybe a day or two more. The fluid will then be reabsorbed but the pain, bruising, and swelling can persist for up to a month.

Possible Complications
Since a very large needle must be used, there's a lot of pain, bruising, and swelling—and all that fluid is reabsorbed within a day. Or, you could get an enormous hematoma if the needle hits a big blood vessel in the breast, or even a whopping infection if any of the bacteria that are normally in the breasts get disrupted. There is also a possibility of an infection, called mastitis, or a blood clot in one of the major blood vessels.

Avoid Being Botched
Why not just put a padded silicone insert in your bra and call it a day?

Science or Scary
A temporary or twenty-four-hour breast lift is touted as an easy way to try out fuller breasts before you go to an event or sign on for implants. The problem is, and the reason I think it's completely bogus, is that you can only inject 200 cc or so of saline and it doesn't simulate breast augmentation very accurately. It's a ridiculous idea, and a very painful one. Do you really want to have terribly sore and discolored and lumpy breasts on your wedding night? You're not going to want your new husband to touch, much less fondle, your breasts because they'll be so swollen and bruised and you'll be in so much agony.

Ultherapy

What It Does

Ultherapy is a noninvasive method of contracting and tightening the loose or sagging skin under the chin.

How It Works

The procedure uses ultrasound to generate a large amount of heat in specific areas, causing thermocoagulation, which makes the skin in the area contract, creating lift.

Lasts For

Depends on the person's features and age. You will see results only after about two to three months once your collagen levels start improving, but it's impossible to predict exact results.

Possible Complications

Redness, swelling, stinging, itching, and bruising. It can also be very, very painful.

Avoid Being Botched

Make sure the device doesn't get anywhere near your eyes.

Science or Scary

This device can penetrate down to your skin's deepest layers, where most of your collagen is found, to stimulate its growth and allow it to reorganize into a more compact and therefore tighter architecture with improved elasticity and firmness. It will never be as effective as a facelift, but some patients do see some firming and lifting of their skin, especially over time as their collagen is stimulated. If you ask most plastic surgeons over cocktails whether Ultherapy really works, they will almost always give a resounding, eh, *kinda*!

Vaginal (and Anal) Steaming

What It Does

Cleanses your vaginal area to improve its health and appearance, and to increase blood flow to the area. Claims are also made that it helps with depression and revitalization.

How It Works

You sit on a sort of throne over an open area of steaming hot, herb-infused vaginal tea.

Lasts For

As long as you're sitting on the throne.

Possible Complications

Burns and irritation; possibly a vaginal infection. Some people, I was told, crank the heat up to ten, but I determined that my pussy is a pussy because I had to turn it all the way down to a three. Because it was *hot*.

Avoid Being Botched

Take a nice hot bath instead. Or find someone with a bidet in their bathroom. The company Toto makes an incredible toilet called the Washlet that has all sorts of adjustable jets. It's heaven for cleansing the area.

Science or Scary

As soon as actress Gwyneth Paltrow claimed on her Goop website that vaginal steaming is "an energetic release—not just a steam douche—that balances female hormone levels," I had to see for myself even though I knew that no steaming can reach your uterus because there's something called a cervix in the way. I found the steaming to be sticky and hot and gross, and then I was informed afterward that I shouldn't be alarmed if I saw any discharge the next day—that it was normal. And that I shouldn't shower for the next day either because I'd get more benefits if I let the herbs sit there. Really? Because when you say *discharge* and *sweaty* I just immediately want to go take a shower. I found the procedure irritating. And as Terry reminded me, the turnover is so fast in the vaginal area, meaning the internal environment is so quickly changed, that any benefits you might get from a steaming are so short lived that it's not worth doing. The only benefit to this procedure was the laughter that ensued from Terry and I making jokes the whole time.

Vaginal Weight Lifting

What It Does

Improves the muscle strength in the pelvic floor and vaginal area.

How It Works

Small weights are inserted in the vagina, and a series of gentle contracting exercises are done to strengthen the muscles.

Lasts For

A while, if you continue doing them.

Possible Complications

Throwing your back out during a class. Or a weight falling on your foot. And . . . what does everyone do with their weights after class? Go to the bathroom and clean them in the sink?

Avoid Being Botched

Yes, there are classes that teach how to do this properly! You need a good instructor to oversee the class.

Science or Scary

Kegel exercises are well known for improving the pelvic floor muscles, and any woman who's done them during pregnancy can vouch for their effectiveness. As women age, too, it is incredibly common to have an overactive bladder, and these exercises are very easy to do and can be a great help. Using weights just ups the training. I personally have no interest in doing this in a group setting. There are better ways to make personal connections—save this one for home!

Whitening Skin Treatments

What It Does

Lightens your skin tone.

How It Works

A stronger concentration of a whitening agent such as hydroquinone or kojic acid is applied during a facial or spa treatment.

Lasts For

It depends on how much of the active ingredient is used, but you won't see much of a difference.

Possible Complications

You can have inflammation, and sometimes, if done with the wrong concentration of active ingredients, the opposite of what you want happens and you get post-inflammatory pigmentation problems, with even more blotchiness.

Avoid Being Botched

Whitening treatments work best, theoretically, on blotchy skin or skin with a lot of hyperpigmentation. Do not expect an esthetician at a spa to be able to treat this. You need a medical professional.

Science or Scary

Wanting to even out your skin tone if it's blotchy and uneven is not the same as wanting to lighten it, of course. Skin whitening has a racial component to it, as some cultures seem to think that the lighter the skin, the better. In South Korea, for example, whitening treatments are pervasive and those with "darker" skin are considered inferior. It's racist and absurd, and it leads women to subject their skin to abuse. Fortunately, the concentration of the lightening agents allowed to be used in spas in America is pretty weak, as otherwise they would be classified as prescription drugs. So at best they'll be barely effective.

◇◇◇◇◇◇◇◇◇◇◇◇◇◇◇◇◇◇◇

As *your* Dr. and Mrs. Guinea Pig, we have tested and shared with you all the best anti-aging information we know. Our hope is that you will use this book as your bible to help you navigate this incredibly confusing world of treatments and procedures. We are here for you, as your friends, and we want to take this anti-aging journey together. Until now, there has been no one guide to help you make a cohesive plan to keep yourself youthful and natural-looking through the decades. I'm lucky to be married to a plastic surgeon who can answer these questions for me—and now you have the power, too! Have fun with this book, and if you have any questions, comments, or suggestions, please reach out to us. We want to hear from you! Twitter and Instagram @heatherdubrow or my website heatherdubrow.com.